This publication offers general insights into the author's family journey through the challenges of cancer and dementia.

Reasonable care has been taken in the preparation of this book and the content is accurate as it relates to the time of the actual events. The author nor the publisher assume any responsibility for errors or omissions. Both parties explicitly disclaim any liability arising from the use or application of the information contained within this book. Furthermore, this content is not intended to provide medical, types of support or other advice suited to individual circumstances. It is solely intended to relay one family's journey and to let others know they are not alone in their struggles.

Copyright © 2025 All rights reserved. No part of this publication may be reproduced, distributed, or transmitted in any form or by any means, including photocopying, recording, or other electronic or mechanical methods, without the prior written permission of the author, except in the case of brief quotations embodied in critical reviews and certain other non-commercial uses permitted by copyright law.

Linda Kaye Randall
LKR Unlimited Opportunities LLC
440 Monticello Avenue STE 1802 #169339
Norfolk, VA 23510-2670

LKR Unlimited Opportunities LLC
Creations Through Grace

Publisher: NewG Praise Productions, LLC

First Edition
ISBN: 979-8-9995168-0-0

Contributing Authors:
Elizabeth J. Randall and Jacqueline A. Weathington

For inquiries about permissions, speaking engagements, or bulk order purchases, please contact linda@lindakayerandall.com

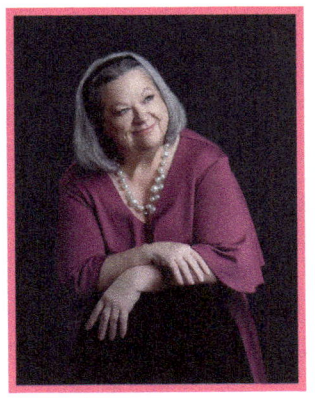

Linda K. Randall, MBA, EMPA
Author & Artist
Linda@lindakayerandall.com

ABOUT THE AUTHOR

Linda Kaye (Carman) Randall grew up in Binghamton, NY. She has two adult daughters, and a dog named Babe. She was with her late husband Gary, the main focus of this book, for twenty-six years. After retiring from a successful Federal Government career, she is now pursuing her passions for writing, painting and spending time with family and friends to make new memories.

She was published in 2024 & 2025 as part of two different anthologies, having successfully launched this book she is already preparing for her next endeavor. All writing and illustrations in this book have been created by the Author, unless otherwise noted.

Follow lindakayerandall.com for what comes next -

Dedications

To my late husband, Gary Lee Bren:

Your life's purpose was to live carefree and to be the rock that allowed us to build a great life. We miss you and this book completes your assignment on earth while you are looking over us from Heaven.

To my daughters, Elizabeth and Jacqueline:

As difficult as our journey was, our Love for Gary and each other, combined with our Faith, allowed us to become stronger, more united and be able to move forward in life with Grace, Compassion and Joy for every moment and each other. God truly blessed us through this journey. Thank you for providing your input into this publication.

To my dear friend, Apostle Andrew L. Campbell:

The Lord spoke through you in 2024 and provided me an opportunity to publish short stories in the Christian anthology, by Dr. Olive C. Brown, called "No Longer in the Waiting Line for Your Promise, Igniting Your Power & Potential". This opportunity provided the confidence to move forward with the vision that was calling me to write about my husband's health journey, which profoundly impacted our family. You have given me non-stop support, prayers and encouragement. Without that this book would likely not exist. I am and will be forever grateful.

To my dear friend, Pamela Goodison:

You have been a continual source of support for me in everything I have accomplished and your support in my endeavors is and will always be greatly appreciated.

To my book coach, Gwen Finley:

You have provided the cloak of accountability I requested to keep me on track as well as becoming a friend and mentor to help frame the vision. You believed in me and encouraged me throughout the process.

To Metropolitan Archbishop Dr. Olive C. Brown:

You provided me the forum to become a publicly published author as well as giving me advice, guidance and continual prayers for the journey.

To my art instructor, Amy Barr:

You have provided ongoing encouragement, support, time, patience and friendship. Your unwavering confidence in my art abilities allowed me to achieve the results I wanted for the illustrations in this book.

My appreciation for having you all in my life can never be fully expressed. You all helped with support, input and accountability of focus –

Thank you!!!

Our collective bond is the commonality of Love, Faith, Frustration, Regret, Pain, Suffering, Anger, Forgiveness, Letting Go, Peace and the ability to Survive.

LKR

1 Peter 4:10 NKJV

As each one has received a gift, minister it to one another, as good stewards of the manifold grace of God.

FOREWORD

There are times in your life when you connect with someone's soul, in an immediate and profound way. These connections may stay for a season, or many, and are filled with deep understanding, authenticity, and vulnerability. Linda is one of these connections for me. We first met in September 2007, both located in Rome, NY for work. She quickly became a close friend and confidant; and we spent the next 5 to 6 years in adjacent cubicles. I have since identified this period in my life as the beginning of a 15-year transformation, filled with many personal growth and development opportunities.

Linda has always been there to listen, and when needed guide, and for this I am forever grateful. Almost 20 years later, we continue our friendship, even though we live in different states. Linda is full of expression, purpose, and always seeking to expand her sense of self, and without a doubt this book is an extension of that, and perhaps just a little bit more.

Just like Linda, the story of her journey with dementia in her family is unforgettable.

Pamela Goodison

FOREWORD

What started as a professional development process turned into a spiritual experience. Linda, I am so Godly proud of this leap of faith in your life. Coming face to face with truth and your willingness to share to help others see that nothing should stop us from reaching our destiny. Though many hurdles, pitfalls and defeats may come our way; however, it is the grace that has been supplied that fuels us in this race. Congratulations and may this writing encourage, strengthen and free others as they read the pages that follow.

++Andrew L Campbell

This Books Framework

There are four main parts to the book:

1. A *narrative section* compiled of chapters touching on specific points of the journey. The goal here is to provide overall context to situations for understanding of impact and to provide knowledge to the reader to help in their journey.

2. *Submissions from the Author's daughters* to provide a glimpse of the impact this journey had on their lives.

3. *Journal Entries* as they were written in date order to provide an in-depth look at the raw personal impact to the family. I allowed this vulnerability in order to provide others the reality of what they may experience and so they do not feel alone. I kept the entries as they related to this particular health journey and did not add input on all the other crazy things that were happening in our world during this timeframe.

4. *A visitation guide* to provide a framework for families to prepare for visits at doctor's offices, treatment sessions and particularly for your time spent with a person dealing with mental decline.

In addition to this book;
A separate companion journal to document your personal journey is also available. It is especially designed to help you easily capture doctor visit notes, thoughts, feelings, etc. for you and/or the afflicted.

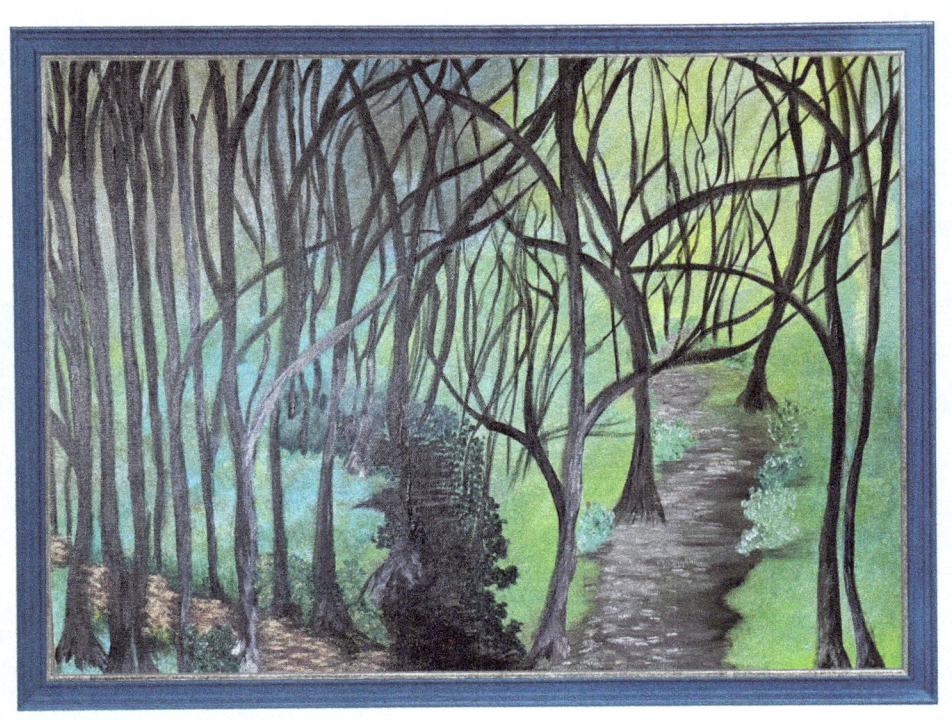

Three Paths Illustration

HABAKKUK 2:2 & 3 (NKJV)

Then the Lord answered me and said:

"Write the vision

And make it plain on tablets,

That he may run who reads it.

For the vision is yet for an appointed time;

But at the end it will speak, and it will not lie.

THE LUMBERJACK SONG

Grace through Hardship

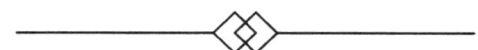

TABLE OF CONTENTS

- Disclaimer
- Introduction
- Random Thoughts

A JOURNEY OF CANCER AND DEMENTIA

1. Lumberjacks
2. The Diagnosis and Decision
3. Chemotherapy
4. Pre-operation Discussions
5. A Journey into Hell
6. Feel What You Feel & Do What You Can Do
7. Things I Never Knew
8. Possessions
9. COVID 19
10. Escape
11. They Are Coming to Get Me – (Rats)

12. The Other Perspective

13. The Calm Before the Storm

14. How Do I Get Out of This?

15. The End of the Winding Road

16. Laying to Rest

DAUGHTERS PERSPECTIVES

Elizabeth (Liz) J. Randall

17. Mind Unraveling, A Heart Breaking

Jacqueline (Jackie) A. (Randall) Weathington

18. Unrecognizable

19. Eulogy for My Father

PERSONAL JOURNAL ENTRIES

- Cancer Treatments
- Post Surgery & Dementia
- Decline and Crossover

VISITATION GUIDE

BLANK NOTE PAGES

DISCLAIMER

THIS BOOK:

IS a real-life account of my family's journey of cancer and dementia.

DOES contain some stories that have literary license applied for effect and they are annotated as such.

IS a story based on actual events and a separate section with specific journal entries that are exact excerpts from what I wrote at the time. These entries provide the emotional aspect of these diseases on families. They are in chronological order and separated by topic for ease of use when reading the story part of the book.

IS intended to be an account of love, advocacy, healing and a test of faith.

IS intended to be a go to publication to help you understand that you are not alone. Although traveling your own specific path the feelings, complexities and impacts are very similar.

DOES allow for an understanding of how to document your journey, make key notes for concerns/questions and memories.

DOES provide specific issues my family encountered with our current health system in order to provide awareness of the importance of independent research, advocacy, and second opinions.

IS NOT intended to advocate for any specific types of treatment, medications, facilities, etc.

IS NOT intended to disparage or undermine our health system or those people who care for others in any way.

DOES NOT contain all the other additional stressors and impacts to families that are thrust upon them daily (job issues, family issues, money, etc.).

DOES NOT offer professional medical advice nor is it to be used in place of professional medical advice.

INTRODUCTION

Inspired by the need to provide insight for people dealing with major health decisions and mental decline, this book is a peak through our window to my family's journey of cancer treatment decisions and their aftermath including vascular dementia. It is **NOT** intended to be a step-by-step decision guide, **NOR** is it intended to say any decision is better than another. These decisions and choices can only be made by the afflicted parties based on their personal needs, desires and resources. The impact on quality of life, family dynamics, caregiving and the healthcare community is profound and worth researching and taking the time to evaluate at the beginning of the journey you are facing.

Based on personal knowledge, actual experiences and time spent interacting with my husband some literary license has been used to capture cohesiveness and to express his "thoughts" when the ability to communicate effectively was impaired. Everyone has to travel their own journey when impacted with life changing events, no two experiences are exactly alike. I hope this book is beneficial as you navigate your journey.

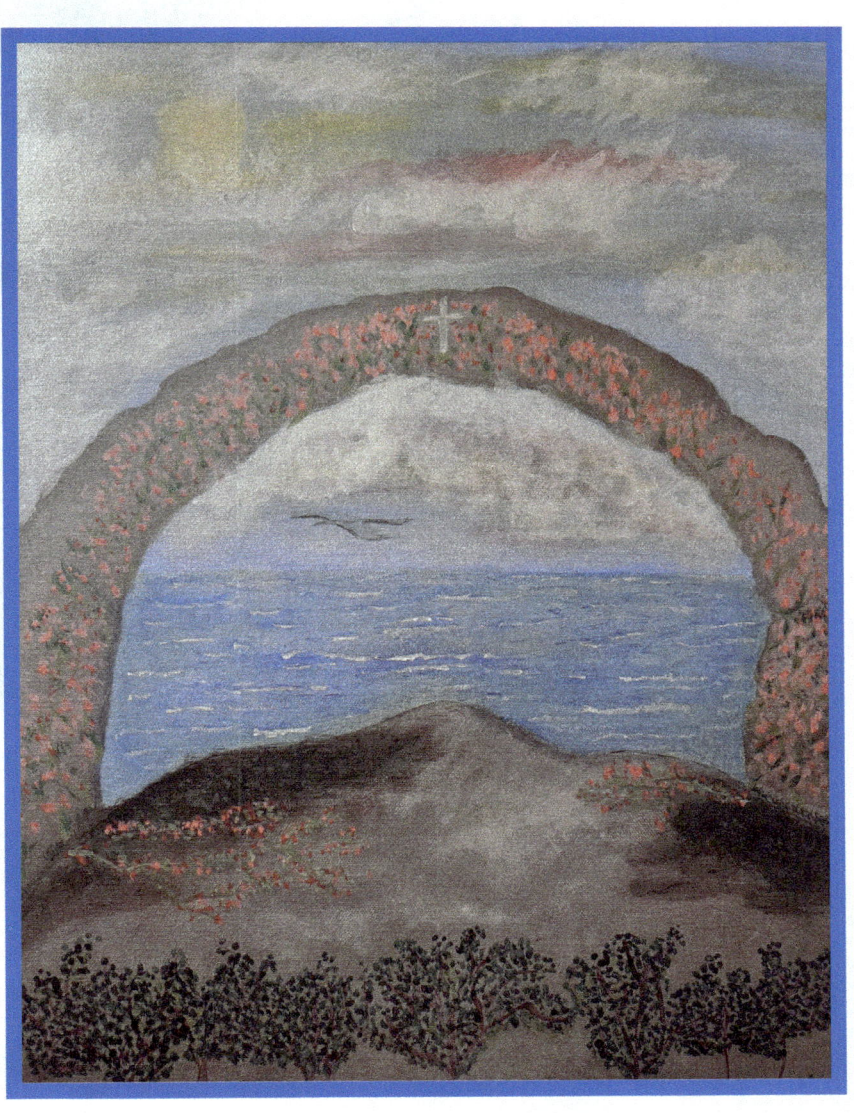

Grace for the Journey

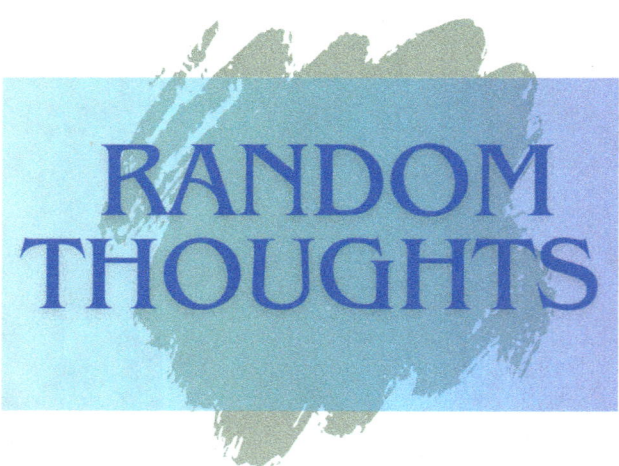

RANDOM THOUGHTS

The process of authoring this book has been daunting. Even though I know it is what I am supposed to do it overtakes me in ways that I cannot fully explain. At times I am able to document things to help other people and at other times it is an emotional and spiritual journey that I have to complete to be truly healed and able to move forward. It is all of these. I find myself wide awake at 4 a.m. or earlier in the morning, thinking about so many things, some pertinent to the book, others just in general of my life with Gary and thinking about what I want for my future. There are days when I am truly happy , but there are times when I feel that something vital is missing. I have worked hard to get myself to a place of having interests outside of the home since retirement and Gary's death, but there is a longing for more. I have grown spiritually, an ever changing process, I have grown emotionally through the grieving process, I have grown physically as I am on an active journey to lose weight by changing my eating and dietary habits and I have grown mentally as I am able to process my triggers and responses with even more clarity. It is a journey of self-discovery, self-love and self-care that I have never gone through before. I have lived my entire life until now in some type of survivor and/or caregiver mode. This change is overwhelming, and I have moments of self-doubt, self-sabotage and wanting to be all alone as well as being with someone.

I have always been a person of faith, however, over the last two years I have with deliberate care been developing a deeper bond with our Lord and Savior, Jesus Christ. I read the Bible, found a Church that I love being part of, was Baptized again and am actively studying the Bible and participating in daily and group prayer. There were, and are, days that include hourly and minute by minute prayers. This has helped guide me on how to move forward with my life.

During and after our family journey with Gary's illnesses I always felt that I would be documenting our trials so that others can have a framework to use in the event they are placed in similar circumstances. I started with a few thoughts but could never get to a point where I could stay focused long enough to finish what I needed to accomplish. Through patience (trust me this is not easy for me), prayer and time to recover emotionally I was able to get clarity of what was holding me back and how to move forward. I realized that I need to have outside parameters to help monitor and control my target milestones. Basically, I needed an invested accountability partner that would collaborate with me on my goals and schedule and help me build an effective schedule with target dates to have things done. Within one week of formalizing this relationship I had already accomplished more than I did in the last eight months.

Life is about understanding yourself, your goals and dreams, writing them down and hopefully with spiritual guidance developing a way forward that is calming, creative and sustainable. There has to be flexibility in this process as we all know Life Happens! When it does, do not get frustrated just adjust your time limits and keep moving forward.

An incredibly special person in my life has really taught me that it is important not to get stuck in whatever Life event you are experiencing, but to gather your spiritual strength in order to move forward. It does not matter if it is a baby step or a running stride, but we have to get up each day and move forward. This does not mean you do not take time to reflect mentally or respond emotionally, but that you get up each day and keep taking care of yourself through proper nutrition, exercise and spiritual focus. Doing this will allow you to stay healthy while you process your mental and emotional well-being.

As I drafted this book, I was mentally reliving the journey, this time with a different perspective, but some days, it was truly exhausting emotionally. I hope that the efforts put forth in this endeavor do help others that are facing severe trials, even if it is only to let them know that they are not alone in their suffering and grief.

God Bless all of you that have taken the time to read this book, fully or piece meal, and I pray for you that you will also have unseen benefits coming forth from the journey.

A JOURNEY OF CANCER AND DEMENTIA

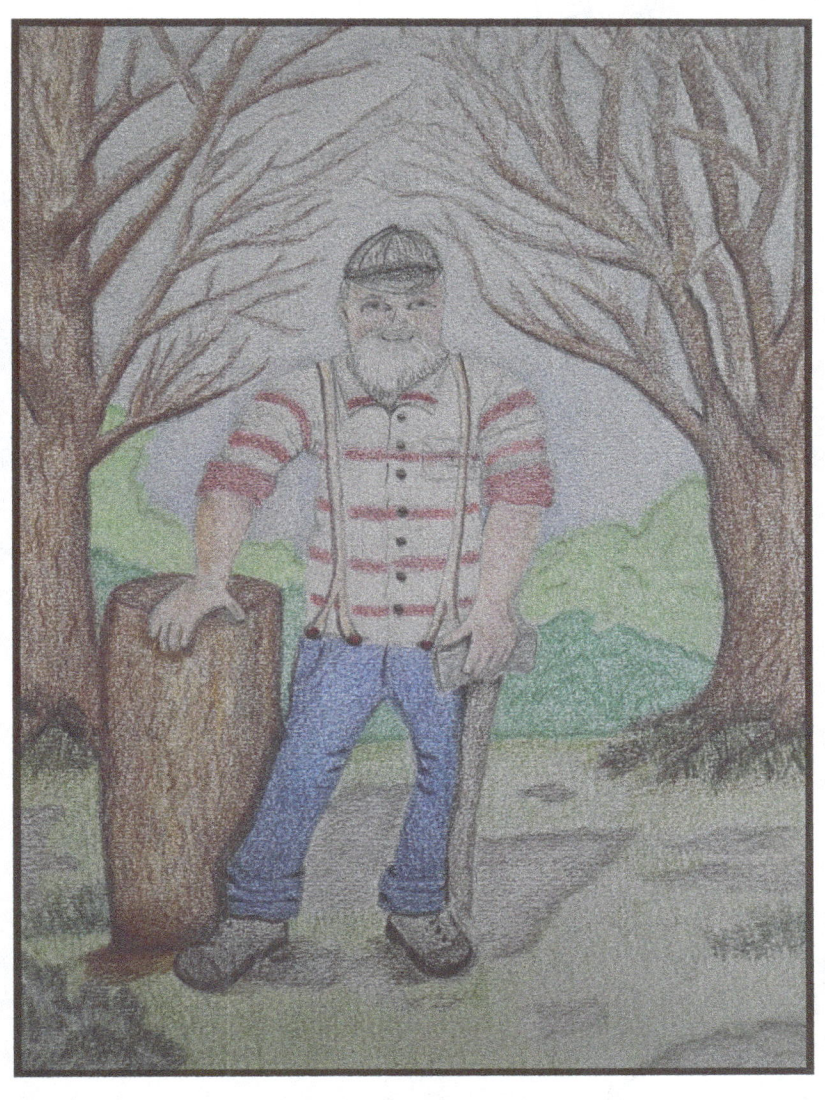

The Lumberjack Song

2 CORINTHIANS 4:16-18

Therefore we do not lose heart.
Even though our outward man is perishing, yet
the inward man is being renewed day by day.

For our light affliction, which is but for a
moment, is working for us a far more exceeding
and eternal weight of glory,
While we do not look at the things which are
seen,
But at the things which are not seen.

For the things which are seen are temporary,
But the things which are not seen are eternal.

Chapter 1

LUMBERJACKS

The sky was crystal blue with a nice breeze and white puffy clouds in the sky. It was turning into a nice early fall day. As I entered the room you could hear humming and the noise of wheels on flooring. I smiled and took a deep breath before I entered the room, maybe it was going to be a good day. The tune was part of one of his favorite songs "I am a Lumberjack and that's o.k."

As I entered the room, he realized I was there and he looked at me with excitement and said to me "Look at how hard they are working" as he turned his gaze to the large bank of windows that overlooked a beautiful tree in the garden visible from his room. The upper half of the tree was visible from the middle of the room and the birds were dancing and singing. Gary was concerned that the lumberjacks were working too hard and that all the trees would be cut down. He pointed out the different men and their ladders, saws and trucks loading up the trunks of the trees. He was mesmerized by the view and told me all the details. I gave him a hug and sat in a chair and let him finish his story. As I listened to the complexities of his current vision of the world, I only saw trees and birds, and I thought to myself there has to be some sense of peace and freedom to be able to live in this alternate version of reality. As he started to wind down his story, I kept it alive by asking him questions about why and what they were working on in order to have some interaction with him. He gladly provided answers with absolute certainty and clarity.

After about an hour he started to become disoriented and asked me how I got there and who I was there to see. Two hours was about the maximum time for a visit as sundowning started settling in early in the day.

I left that day with a sense of peace that at least for those two hours we had a great time together and shared something very unique.

For those that may not currently be familiar with sundowning, it is the point at which individuals with memory disorders start to really have trouble tracking, remembering and being able to annunciate properly for communication. The physical disability of their disease takes over any conscious desire of what they want to relay. As the disease progresses this period of the day gets earlier and earlier and depending on the physical longevity can be permanent with the afflicted being unable to communicate or do anything physical on their own. Heartbreaking to watch.

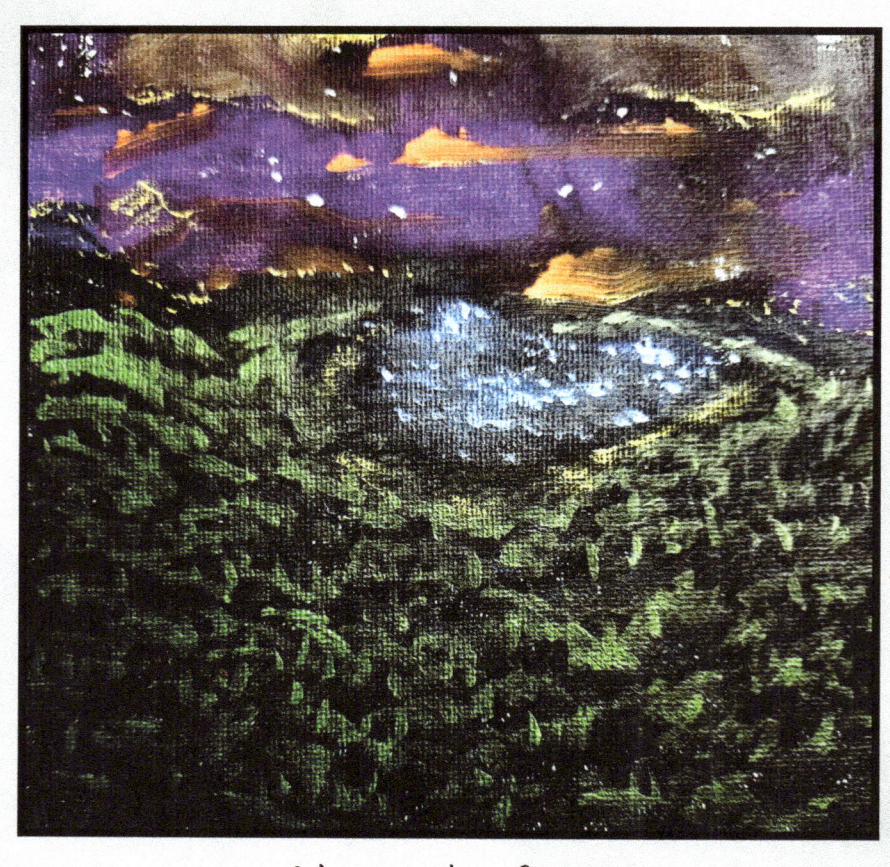

Nature's Unrest

JAMES 5:15 NKJV

And the prayer of faith will save the sick, and the Lord will raise him up.

And if he has committed sins, he will be forgiven.

Chapter 2

THE DIAGNOSIS AND DECISION

The sun had been shining upon our home for two months after receiving the news that Gary's cancer had been cured. We were very thankful and had started to rejoice in the possibilities for the summer and years ahead. We had not been in our new home long when he was diagnosed so we had not had a chance to enjoy all that was available to us in our new location. We started to discuss what activities we would like to do together when I wasn't working and he would continue to enjoy riding his motorcycle when I was not at home.

The first week of June was upon us and Gary needed to have a follow-up visit. We were very hopeful as we went into the Doctor's office as we were told previously that the cancer was gone. It was considered a common treatable cancer with a low recidivism rate. The exam for bladder cancer is an invasive test that is painful, and it made me feel very empathetic for Gary as I could only imagine what he felt from a pride and pain standpoint. As I watched my husband undergo yet another procedure, I prayed that it would be over, so he didn't have to undergo this anymore. Life had other things in store for us. The Doctor said he would have to undergo another bladder biopsy as he spotted a new spot on his bladder. The sun had turned into darkness again as we listened and postured for yet another test.

The biopsy was performed very soon after the exam and the results were that Gary had an extremely rare and aggressive small cell carcinoma cancer of the bladder. It was in the early stages and without treatment Gary had about fifteen to eighteen months to live. With aggressive chemotherapy and surgery to remove his bladder and prostate he had a chance to live at least five years. This cancer type is so rare that there is no established treatment plan or survival statistics post treatment. We were hoping for the best. Gary's health and age would be a major factor in the outcome of any treatment.

Gary being fifteen years my senior had never really played much into our relationship as he had always been a very vibrant, fun and active man. The last year had been filled with multiple health issues for both of us and the first cancer diagnosis placed me in a major caregiver/survivor mode that shut off emotions in order to function on a daily basis. Gary had to concentrate on his will and faith that he would get through the treatments and be cured. These singular focuses guided our discussions to topics surrounding care and forward planning. I would cry in private and had to remain strong for Gary and for my daughters so that they would not have to carry any of the day-to-day burdens.

This new diagnosis rocked our world in a way that is hard to describe. Our ability to remain positive was tested as being the practical realists we had to discuss in detail topics of death, estate plans, funeral and burial arrangements, long term care, etc. This was physically and emotionally exhausting by itself, let alone dealing with the actual treatment plans and impacts. I felt my world falling apart and Gary who normally was a quiet man opened up about how petrified he was of what would happen and how it would impact our life together.

To know Gary is to understand that he was a strong independent man that loved his family. God brought Gary into my life after my previous marriage of fifteen years ended in divorce. When we met my daughters were almost six and just over two years old. When I realized that I wanted to pursue a relationship with Gary he was introduced to my daughters and there was instant love all around as they adored him, he them, and Gary and I fell so in love it was incredible. Soon after we were a family, traveling and living all over the world, experiencing life to the fullest. Gary loved music and one of his favorite songs to sing was the version of the "Lumberjack Song" by Monty Python. It made all of us laugh and being from Minnesota where the eighteen foot lumberjack statue of Paul Bunyan resides made it special to him, and he took us to see the statue.

When Gary received this second cancer diagnosis our daughters were on their own as we were in our twenty-second year together with nineteen of those being married. Even though I was still working I was getting closer to the point I could retire, so we could do things together anytime. We both felt that our good days were behind us and we had instantly entered into the last phase of life.

It was time for a decision. Would Gary undergo aggressive chemotherapy and surgery or would Gary live life to the fullest on whatever time the cancer gave him? It is incredibly hard not to be selfish during these types of decisions, but it had to be up to Gary to decide how to live out the rest of his life and I would be his advocate for whatever decision he made. Being a Virgo I am an excellent researcher, question asker, organizer and planner so once decided the best way forward would be analyzed and executed. He decided to proceed with the treatment plan. I believe in my heart today that Gary loved his family so much that he wanted to try to survive and live and did not really understand or comprehend the impacts chemo and surgery would have on his overall quality of life.

Note: Always research information extensively on impacts to quality of life from various sources, not just Doctors. Doctors want to save a life, but they are not your advocate as to how well you live your life, statistics of avoiding death are what matter to them. You have to be assertive, ask questions and insist that they do as you wish.

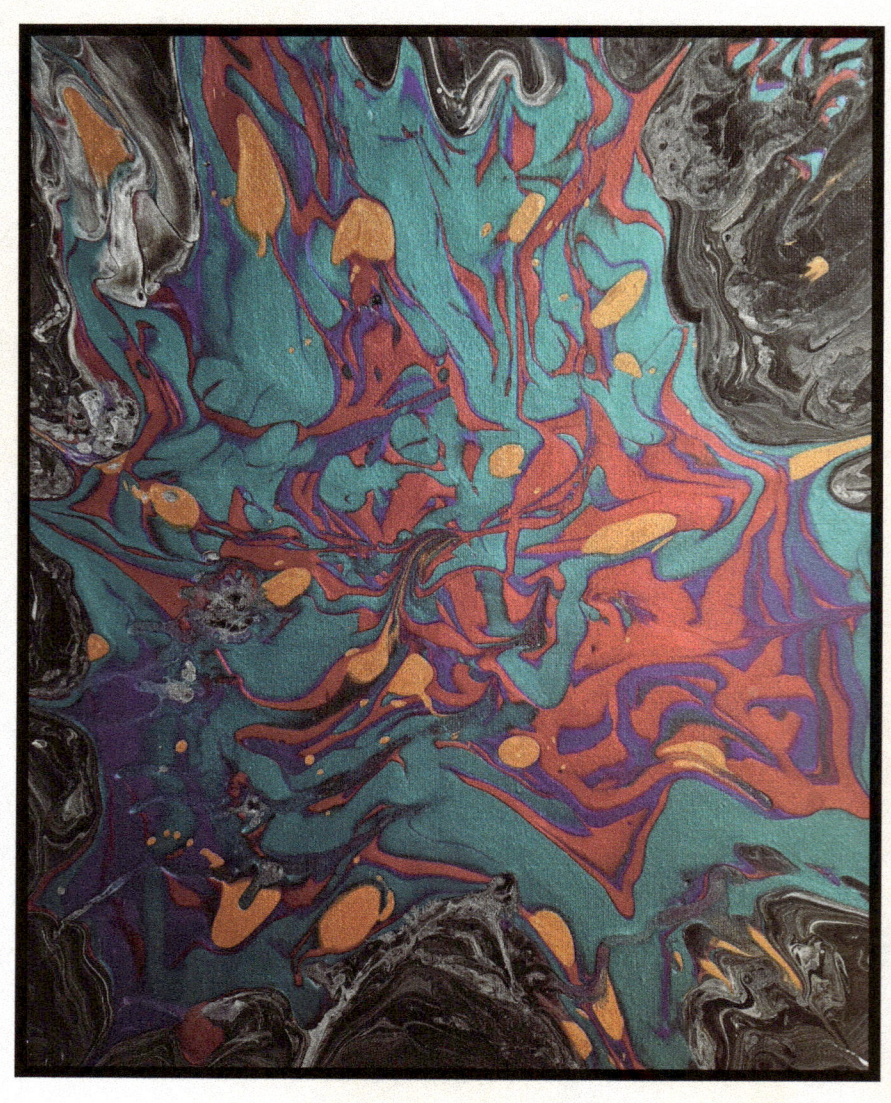

Angels & Demons

Chapter 3

CHEMOTHERAPY

Once the decisions were made chemotherapy treatment started. Regardless of what the Doctor's tell you about the therapy anticipate the worst scenario, then you will be more prepared than if you only consider the best. This is not to say do not be hopeful for a cure, but to anticipate that the treatment itself could be the hardest with the most side effects in order to mentally prepare you and your family. Being hopeful people, we went into this armed with answers to so many questions the doctor was overwhelmed.

Every treatment with chemotherapy is specially designed for each person's medical diagnosis and their body. For Gary this meant four rounds of a special blend of chemotherapy drugs. A round of chemotherapy is not the number of bags or visits; it is what is considered the amount required to have an impact on the cancer in progressive stages to achieve optimal results. In Gary's situation this meant four rounds with each round consisting of three days in a week receiving various types and amounts of cell destroying drugs and twenty-one days before the next three-day cycle. The hope is to kill more cancer cells than normal ones. Gary had to undergo an eight-hour treatment for the first day which involved receiving three bags total of two different types of chemo drugs. This was followed by two days of receiving one to two bags of one of the chemo drugs based on blood work results with each session lasting three to five hours.

In addition, bags of fluid have to be pumped into the patient to prevent kidney damage at each visit. That was considered one round. In twenty-one days, he would receive round two, then twenty-one days later round three, etc. for a total of four rounds. The entire process would last over two and half months.

Even with all the information you can never be fully prepared and especially when you have to balance work, caregiving and the will of a strong husband. One of the things you are told is that the physical impacts of chemo will hit you about two to three days after the treatment and you will start to feel better right before you start the next treatment. Wonderful way to anticipate your days. This is also dependent on the individual and chemo dosage, the doctors do not know how it will impact you until it does, so be honest and forthright about how it impacts you. Gary's cancer being so aggressive required a strong plan that included two different types of chemo drugs forced in during the course of a week. Just about the time the first session was impacting the second session was in play.

Gary insisted that I go to work and at the time I was not allowed to work from home and care for Gary, so to work I went. Anyone in this situation understands how quickly your leave gets used when you have ongoing health concerns.

Gary was that husband that always greeted you when you came home, he was already retired when his illness took over. Upon coming into the driveway after work about a week after the first week of chemo Gary greeted me on the porch. Gary was a very meticulous man. He was a casual dresser, jeans, button down shirt or T-Shirt with work boots, but he was always groomed well and did not wear summer clothes. It was July and upon my arrival I was greeted with a man only in his underwear and on his left foot he had on a sock and shoe and was barefoot on the other foot. I looked at Gary and thought to myself "What is going on, what am I getting into?" As I got out of the car, I asked him why he was on the porch in his underwear, and he just looked at me with a confused expression and said, "I don't know what's happening." My emergency response kicked in as I was trying to assess what was happening. I saw the confusion and fear in Gary's face and his voice was disjointed, quivering and soft as he responded that he did not know what was going on.

He was able to walk with assistance, so I got him into the house, to his chair and told him not to get up. He acted drunk, but I knew that it had to be a chemo reaction. I started to look for his clothes, shoes and wallet, they were scattered all over the house. The man must have been removing stuff at various points in his journey through the house. I called my neighbor to come help me as I knew given his condition, I could not get him dressed by myself to get him to the ER. He did not want to go so an ambulance was not the best solution. After finding his wallet with his insurance cards and ID buried in the bed under the blankets, we were able to get him into the car and my neighbor drove us to the ER.

The chemo had totally annihilated all of his immune system and he had a major infection. He ended up in the hospital for a week. The doctor said if we wait for him to fully recover then he would have to start the cycle of treatments from the beginning. That was not an option Gary was willing to do (understandably). At the beginning of the next week, he was back at treatment with the dosage adjusted based on what happened. We discussed whether or not he wanted to continue the therapy and he said, "I've decided to do it, so I will continue." He managed the remaining chemo treatments better, but you could see how weak and frail he was becoming. The infection could have been a factor in his brain deterioration, but was not identified at the time, as chemo brain fog is a known side effect of chemotherapy.

He wanted desperately to go on motorcycle rides and he even put on his helmet one day to do just that as he was feeling a bit better towards the end of one the cycles, but I had to take away the keys as he was not strong or agile and I feared that he could hurt others as well as himself. I believe he may have wanted to just take himself out with a good ride, but unfortunately for him I intervened.

There is always a positive out of every negative situation. The chemo sessions were a bonding experience for Gary and me as well as getting to know some incredibly special people that were going through their own struggles. The nurses are exceptional people and unbelievably we found ways to smile and laugh while attending the sessions. You absolutely reaffirm what is really important in life when you experience these tests.

Chapter 4

PRE- OPERATION DISCUSSIONS

As my husband became weaker and lost his hair from chemotherapy it was time to start having the discussions of the surgery procedure, impacts to quality of life and any verified statistics on life expectancy. As a detail fact-oriented type personality, as well as being my husband's medical advocate, many hours of research were completed prior to meeting with the surgeon. When I say many hours, at least forty hours researching, reading and writing down questions and concerns. Then researching more to find those answers prior to meeting with the surgeon. His cancer was so rare and the procedure was still relatively new in helping to remove any chance of recurrence that getting information proved exceedingly difficult. At the time of his cancer and surgery he would be one of a handful of people with this type of cancer and there were very few medical statistics on effectiveness, prognosis and results over a five-year period. That was just the cancer, let alone there were no statistics on what impact the procedure would have on the cancer or quality of life. What I did find did not paint a good picture as most of the patients with this cancer regardless of treatment did not survive past twenty four months and none had survived at the five year point.

The surgeon was a urologist and was collaborating with the oncologist on what the cancer status was for my husband. As all surgeons tend to be, they are a bit on the pompous side and do not like being questioned or called out when something they say does not correlate with the research brought to them by patients or advocates.

Even though he realized that I came armed to have answers, he was not really prepared to provide answers to many of the questions, especially quality of life concerns. He just said that patients he had so far had no issues taking care of their bag changes themselves. The surgeon did not concern himself with Gary's age or the impacts that Chemo and the infections may have already had on his body. No mention of doing an extensive memory test to see if he had any other underlying issues. He did not bother to relate to the fact that Gary was not currently functioning at full capacity and when asked about what was entailed in the daily care of the ileostomy, he just relayed that the nurses would train us to do it. This did not provide a sense of reassurance and in fact made me angry. I honestly believe that he had no idea what the daily care routine would require and we both felt that he had no compassion. There were not a lot of surgeons that could perform this particular surgery at the time, so I had to remain constrained in my responses, but continued to ask questions and make notes. He was to undergo an ileostomy which would remove the bladder and prostrate and create a stoma on the right side of his small intestine, which would always have a bag attached to it, as all control of urinary function would be gone. After much discussion Gary decided to have the surgery as "I have already gone this far, I need to go the full distance."

Note: A Surgeon's livelihood is based on how many successful surgeries they perform, no real consideration is given to patients' impacts after the surgery – just that the specific procedure they are to perform goes well and the patient survives the operation. Once the surgery itself is considered successful they are out of your lives forever. The onus of any lingering after surgery concerns and care are thrust upon the rest of the medical community and family whether or not they have any understanding of the impacts from the surgery or proper training on new procedures. Keep in mind, given their limited visibility on the patient most surgeons have no idea what quality life impacts really exist, method or extent of care needed or long-term impacts, so they are not in a position to provide any qualified credible guidance in this area. If a procedure is routine, it is easy to find others to get information from, but when a procedure is relatively rare or new there is no one to reach out to and the medical support community may not be postured to provide what is necessary. This is what happened to us.

Chapter 5

JOURNEY INTO HELL

The day of the surgery arrived. We were ready. Early arrival at the hospital to ensure that all pre-operative procedures took place and to be attentive to Gary and the doctors as they brought any last-minute information to the table. Nervous, hopeful, and prayer filled for what we anticipated to be a good outcome.

After all the nurses and the surgeon did their things, we were still of the same mindset. Then came the anesthesiologist and his assistant. They reviewed Gary's history, looked at him and dropped the bombshell. Given Gary's history with the chemotherapy, infections, his heart and his age he was extremely concerned that the surgery being very lengthy would have a negative impact on his outcome. He said that they would attempt to keep him at the lowest dosage possible and would use the anesthesia that would have the least chance of negatively impacting him.

At that point, the world stopped. Talk about having to make a major decision in a short period of time. He literally was moments away from being wheeled into the operating room. We asked for a few minutes alone to make the decision and the anesthesiologist was genuinely nice and agreed we needed to take some time. Once alone we talked about how this was never discussed as part of the treatment or surgery discussions and that if it had been it likely would have changed the entire course of his treatment journey.

We all looked at each other and then asked Gary what he wanted to do. Gary took a few deep breaths and then looked at us and said that he had mentally prepared for the surgery and at this point he may as well go ahead with it. The decision was made; it was his to make.

We hugged, kissed, expressed our love for one another and prayed. They rolled Gary away; we all had quivering smiles and tears as he left our sight. That was the last time we saw the husband and father of our family as the man he always was, a boulder of strength, a whole person.

The next month was a horror that I would not wish on my worst enemy. Gary had a negative reaction to the anesthesia and he was out of his mind after the surgery. He had no idea what had happened to him, where he was and was very distraught. The hospital had to constrain him to keep him from pulling at his ileostomy as well to prevent him from getting up out of the bed. He had to be sedated but the level of sedation had to be limited as he had to get healed and be mobile to allow for the procedure to work properly. He yelled and screamed at everyone, he didn't understand and based on the discussions with the doctors he likely would never be the same. He had to have CNAs come in to sit with him to keep him calm when we were not there.

The nurses and I had to learn how to change his bag and clean the wound. The majority of the nurses, to include the RNs, had no idea how to deal with this type of wound care.

Gary would require rehabilitation in a skilled nursing facility (SNF) which hopefully would allow him to regain some physical and mental capabilities through ongoing therapies. In order for that to happen he had to be unconstrained without a sitter for twenty-four hours - that in itself was a major challenge and required the nurses to constantly be coming by his room to check on him. They were all worn out and ready to transfer him to a different level of care, because the hospital couldn't really do anything for him.

Finally, the day came he could be transferred. We had visited and selected a place near the hospital that appeared to be better than other options we visited. Appearances are deceiving and keep in mind that our health care system has been in crisis for a while with staffing issues. He was placed when a room became available. His room was at the end of a hallway near an exit door.

This particular place was a horror show due to inadequate staffing and the inability of the staff to manage this type of wound. We had to almost beg for them to take Gary to begin with as other places were so bad or flat out refused to be burdened with Gary's unique care situation with the ileostomy. Due to Gary's unique surgery and his current physical and mental issues, the staff was not able to keep up with his needs. Elizabeth ended up having to stay with him overnight to keep him calm as he would try and get up, pull out his bag, make a mess and almost fall without constant supervision. She even had to help get him to the bathroom and provide full caregiver needs as the staff were both untrained and had too many residents to properly care for him. This burden fell on me during the days, and my sister and Jackie would also provide relief as they could. At one point I had to take over the night shift as Elizabeth was at her limit – completely understandable.

This narrative does not fully describe the absolute hellish period of his SNF experience. After a discussion with the Head of Nursing and the other board members they did feel that they could not do anything more for Gary. He had gotten a bit better with his therapy sessions, but he needed to be somewhere where he could receive more one-to-one care. They were willing to keep him until the 100 days under Medicare ran out, but we would still have to provide 24-hour supervision.

My thoughts on this were, if we have to be the ones doing the work, why am I paying this facility? The point was noted, and the Head nurse was able to have a private discussion with me regarding a small group home assisted living facility that specialized in residents with memory issues. We set up an appointment.

This is another point in my life where I knew with absolute certainty that the Grace of God was looking over us. Two of the most wonderful people I have ever met came to the SNF to meet us. After seeing Gary and assessing his care needs, they said they had room and could take Gary. She was going to get training for her and all the staff to be able to properly take care of his ileostomy needs, he would have therapy sessions and he would start to thrive in a homey environment.

She was absolutely correct. Even though there was no chance of him ever coming home and he would continue to decline over time he was able to be calm, have his needs met, and regain his ability to walk and do stairs for a period of time. He liked it there, he had a fenced yard with a complicated lock to walk in (he figured out how to work it), excellent food – he gained some weight back – and liked the staff. We were able to have nice visits.

Over time as his health declined, he was transitioned to a full memory care facility that was locked down. He missed his freedom.

***NOTE:** When discussing treatment and outcomes, you need to look from beginning to end and ask additional questions as events occur. Even though I asked questions about his condition and the surgery the anesthesiologist was never fully consulted by the surgeon, oncologist, primary doctor or urologist prior to the day of the surgery. I also don't believe based on our experience that any conversations occurred prior to the day of the surgery, little to no consideration of whether a person can manage what they suggest.*

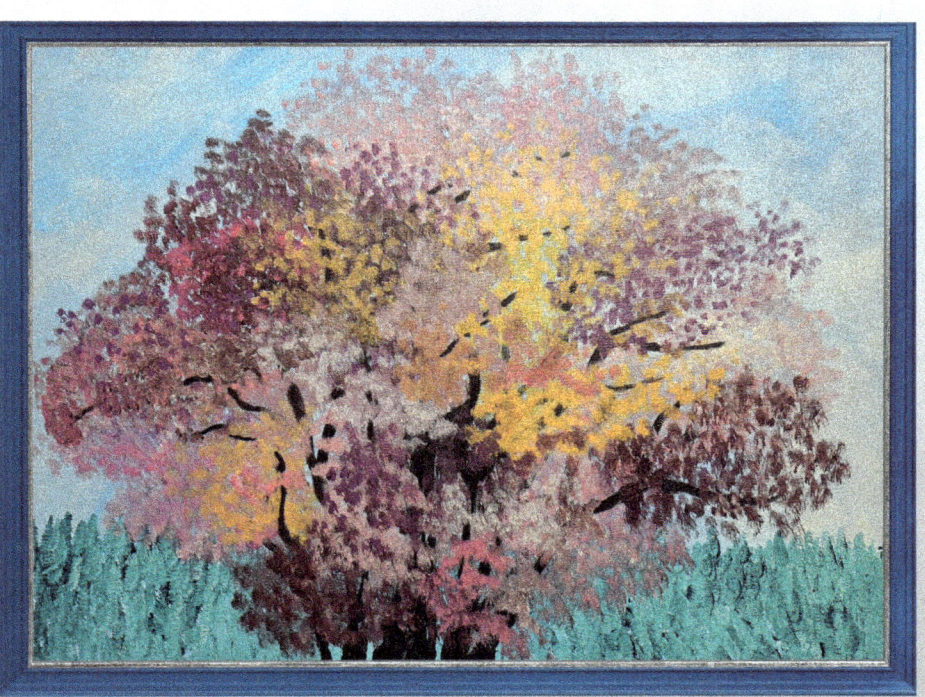

Fifty Fruit Tree

PHILIPPIANS 2:27 NKJV

For indeed he was sick almost unto death:

But God had mercy on him,

And not only on him but on me also,

Lest I should have sorrow upon sorrow.

Chapter 6

FEEL WHAT YOU FEEL & DO WHAT YOU CAN DO

It is amazing to me that so many people, to include myself at times, are ashamed at the emotions that they have during different situations. We are human beings, not robots, it is o.k. to feel. In fact, our ability to feel a wide range of emotions sets us apart from the other living creatures on the planet and is a gift from our creator. Anyone going through crisis, long term illness and grief and loss should be dealing with a wide range of emotional upheaval or there may be larger concerns at play. Yes, it is true that if you are a believer, you are able to trust in God, but part of that is allowing yourself to free yourself of whatever human feelings overtake you. Cry, scream, write, throw things (carefully), break things, sleep, meditate, exercise, eat well, drink water and pray with all your might. It is important to do these things in your private space and not while you are on a visit. Constant awareness of clarity of the person afflicted is essential when wanting to express any emotions, they may not understand what is happening or why.

I am here to tell you that as you are embarking on a journey of long-term illness and/or dementia-related diseases it may be the hardest thing you will ever have to suffer. This is not only true for the patient, but for anyone who loves the person that is afflicted. There is no one way to deal with the process as every single journey will be different. You and your loved ones are in fact dealing with grief and loss, just as if someone has already died, but with no immediate closure. Each day takes a piece of your heart and the hopes for your future life away from you and what is left is uncertainty and pain of living through an extended period of gradual loss of your loved one.

Unfortunately, there is also for far too many people a major financial upheaval that occurs in these situations as well. The availability of Long-Term Care Insurance is not something most people have the luxury of affording or even realize it is available. A hint is that if you are able to work it within your budget do it as early as possible, the younger you are the cheaper your premiums are for life. Anyway, not to sidetrack, the bulk of people even with LTC Ins will have to outlay at least 90 days' worth of expenses for health care for afflicted parties if they do not have enough family help during these times. It is expensive, so debt can very quickly become an additional burden.

With all of this the range of emotions will be all over the place and not everyone will be feeling the same emotions at the same time. There will likely be anger, denial, disbelief, profound sadness, regret, loneliness, sleep deprivation, nightmares, resentment, major decisions to be made, support systems to develop, financial uncertainty, frustration and a necessity to learn a lot quickly all before you are able to reach a place of acceptance and security knowing your loved one is being cared for in the best manner you are able to provide. That sounds extremely daunting, and it is, even when you have planned for such things. Most of the same range of emotions are being experienced by the afflicted as well. It is important to understand the patient's current level of understanding to determine the extent of what is shared as it relates to care, family issues, worldly issues and the issues that surround them. Stressful conversations are not good for those with memory issues, they get confused, stressed and it may trigger frustration when they see their loved ones upset.

It is essential that you and any loved ones, progress through this journey with a safe space to express yourself. This includes support groups or other people you are close to that have experienced a similar journey. If someone has not experienced it, they are not fully engaged in your support, because they cannot fully relate to your experience, no matter how much they want to help. This also includes a safe place to isolate and regain control over your emotions and thoughts. Try not to converse with anyone when you are not in control of your emotions, it will lead to discord and potentially detrimental consequences. Discuss matters as they arise when people have calmed down and are ready to have mature conversations. Age and mental state have to be considered in how and when to approach issues.

Everyone has to determine the level of support they are able to provide for their loved ones, this is as unique as you are as a person. I do know that unless you have help trying to do everything yourself can be a major problem as you may not have the mental or physical stamina required to provide the proper care. Really take the time to evaluate your path forward. Remember the initial decision does not have to be permanent in a lot of cases. Life can allow you to change your mind in order to provide yourself with self-care.

Chapter 7

THINGS I NEVER KNEW

It is fascinating that after being together for twenty-three years before his dementia set in how much you still do not know about a person. We get so busy with everyday life and the comfort of just being that unless something specifically prompts a question or conversation, there is not that much inquiry that still takes place about each other. Love has a way of not requiring additional knowledge after you know that trust, friendship, respect and loyalty are what you have with each other.

In our family's dementia journey together, we learned a lot about each other and ourselves. As each visit unfolded there was always anticipation of whether there would be silence, laughter, crying, disappointment, anger, fear or pure love. It is necessary to prepare yourself prior to visits with your loved ones to expect the unexpected and be thankful for the days that are calm or bring special joy.

In an effort to try and prolong Gary's memory the family prepared several memory books. Please note that these things need to be brought with you each visit to avoid any damage or misplacement These memory books play a vital role in helping dementia patients to remember who people are and what period they are living in.

In addition, this is where a wealth of information from Gary's life before I met him came flowing to the surface. His sister had created a family history album, and it contained the names and dates of many events in Gary's past. When I took this in on several occasions, we were able to look at the pictures and I had Gary tell me stories about the time and people in the pictures. I would document what he relayed to me, so that we could have that for our next time revisiting the books. This was good for him, because it kept his brain active, dementia patients lose recent memories first, so he was able to really capture those memories from long ago. I learned so much from his childhood that he never talked about before that I felt I was really starting to understand more of what made my husband the man he had become.

He was able to let go of inhibitions when telling stories, because the part of the brain that creates barriers is not as active as a patient declines. This allowed him to fully express his emotions based on certain events and allow a connection to me that we never experienced before. Full transparency dictates that I say be prepared for anything, not everyone's past experiences are all roses and sunshine and can truly be heartbreaking.

Most of the time he was able to laugh and rejoice in talking about how he picked on his little sister or the dinner competitions with his brother to get to the last piece of meat or potatoes on the dinner table, often involving the possibility of getting stabbed with a knife. There were even memories of his first kiss with a sweet little girl when he was just a little boy. I absorbed these discussions as I knew that my time to get to know him at this level was getting shorter by the day. Did I reciprocate with the same types of memories, not unless specifically asked, because it would be a present conversation that he would not remember in a few hours or create confusion thinking it happened recently possibly creating trauma for him.

As stated previously it is important to remain flexible with your expectations as over the course of a one to two-hour visit there can be many moods, level of engagement and physical activity. These visits are so important; however, they are truly mentally and physically exhausting for the survivor as well as the patient. I would be completely drained at the end of the visit with no capability to do anything else for the day. My day usually ended with a mid-afternoon nap.

I alternated the books between recent, recent past to older to get a status check on his memory capabilities from week to week. Some days they did not come out of my bag as he would not be able to focus, or he was lost in his own world. Those days were hard. The hardest day was when I entered the room and his memory was so far back that he thought I was his mother. That day he really did not know who I was, so holding back tears I put on a smile and went back in time to the world he was living in and conversed with him as though I was his mom. This made him happy, and he talked about the cow he had on the farm and that he needed to go out and milk it, so they had fresh milk for dinner. That day I knew that I had really lost my husband and now we were just in a vicious cycle of testing and trial (otherwise known as prison) with no set date of release. I cried and prayed for strength for days until I was able to regain the courage to go back to visit.

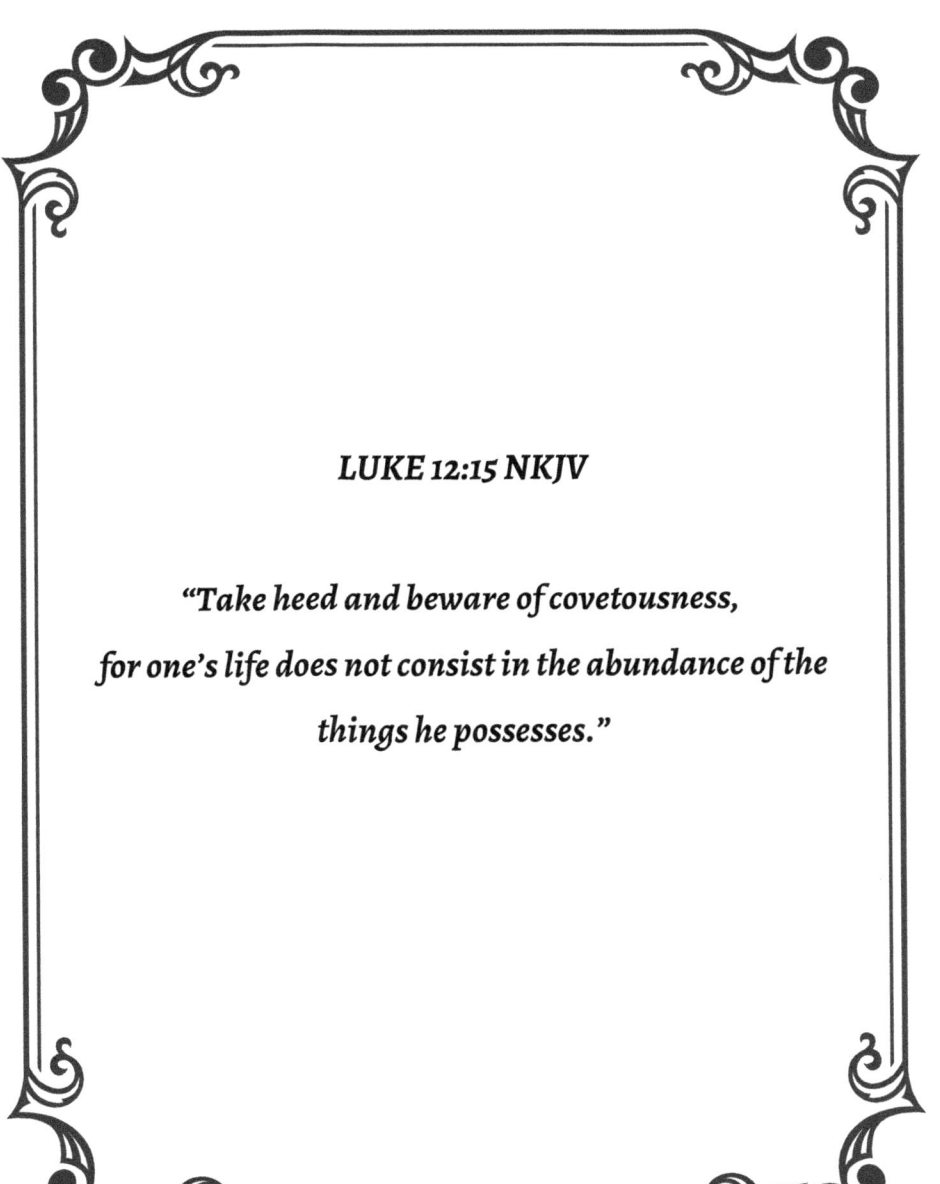

LUKE 12:15 NKJV

"Take heed and beware of covetousness, for one's life does not consist in the abundance of the things he possesses."

Chapter 8

POSSESSIONS

What material possessions do you covet the most? This is a particularly important question. We all recognize that material possessions do not come with us when we pass over, however, we still desire them. Each one of us has a different level of material desire and different things that are important to us. Most of us have far too many things that hold little or no meaning other than to decorate a living space that is more than we need to occupy. I want you to take the time to really assess the top ten to twenty possessions that have the most emotional impact to your well-being. This is not money, important papers, clothing, furniture or necessarily high value items, but those things that you have held on to that bring you peace or evoke a series of happy memories for you when you touch or look at them.

Once you have thought about this, document this on paper in a safe place for your loved ones or care givers. These are the items you will want in the event you are required to have full- time care and be in a confined living space. You will want to ensure that you have things that bring you peace. In addition, write down those things that you like to do; hobbies, activities, social events, etc. This information is valuable to ensure if you are not able to speak for yourself others can speak accurately for you. We are talking about your ability to adapt and transition with your situation as life's journey unfolds.

Care giving facilities in general do not have large spaces and often have special restrictions as to the amount, type, size and placement of items that can be brought with you. In addition, depending on your situation you may be sharing a room, needing room space for medical equipment and supplies, limiting these items even further.

In my experience, you want to ensure a familiar comfortable space while maintaining space to roam, especially for dementia patients that still have mobility in any capacity. Avoid any items that can create a state of mental stimulation that creates confusion or images that may spark delusions (many abstract art pieces). Pictures with familiar faces are great as it helps to prolong the recognition of loved ones (put names on the photos to help memory association with who they are to you). Items from favorite places and events help stimulate conversation during visits and testing what period the mind is focusing on. It is okay to switch out items one at a time but be sure that the patient is engaged in the process. If the person is no longer able to provide permission in a lucid moment, keep things the same to avoid confusion and frustration thinking something has been taken from them when you are not there to reassure them.

Also, keep in mind that things can disappear from the room. This is not usually a "theft," but a replacement of items. This can occur by the patient not realizing where or who they gave things to as well as staff, particularly when it comes to clothing – even items with proper labeling get reassigned temporarily due to volume and lack of staffing. Go into the situation realizing things are going to happen, so don't take family heirlooms/special keepsakes in there if you aren't willing to risk breakage or loss.

My husband had angry, frustrating episodes that were so out of his normal behavior, and he would break, throw and take apart things a lot. His laundry was always in a state of crazy, simply because he went through multiple sets of clothing a day due to him pulling on his ileostomy bag and he would constantly be rearranging his items, so no one knew where anything was located. Clothing needs should be discussed with the facility based on the patients' needs. This may dictate a whole change in how a person normally clothes themselves. My husband had to go from a man that wore work boots, jeans, tucked in button down or T-shirts to sweatpants and very loose pull over T-shirts with slip on shoes. This was very distressing at first for him, until he decided they were in fact comfortable.

Please be kind to the staff and caregivers, they are all overworked and underpaid and have their primary focus on the physical well-being of your loved one, not their possessions.

MATTHEW 11:28-29 NKJV

Come to Me, all you who labor and are heavy laden,
And I will give you rest.
Take My yoke upon you and learn from Me,
For I am gentle and lowly in heart,
And you will find rest for your souls.

Chapter 9

COVID 19

As my husband transitioned from a skilled nursing facility to the assisted living group home for memory care patients in late January 2020, the world was starting to hear about COVID 19 and the possible devastation that could happen if it became a worldwide pandemic. The concern was real and in early January I had already started to build a small supply of canned goods and non-perishable items to have on hand. Not being a hoarder and being aware of other people's needs I was not someone that bought a bunch of toilet paper, etc. as I just anticipated a month or two of what I would need. Looking back, I was thankful God gave me the grace to plan ahead - who knew how crazy it would get. Anyway, Gary at this point was just getting used to his new home and his fellow housemates. I thanked God every day that He brought us to this small group home as it really helped with his transition away from home. Being an actual home, he was able to have a cozy environment with an enclosed yard to walk in and he had full-time care with a personal touch due to the caregiver-to-patient ratio. It was only a few weeks after he moved in that all nursing homes and assisted facilities had to close their doors to visitors. This was devastating to everyone not to be able to see those you love.

This was very upsetting to me, but I was able to call Gary and talk to him for a few minutes whenever I wanted to so that was immensely helpful. What was an unexpected blessing from this was that the forced separation provided a guilt free way of adjusting to the new life that both of us were embarking on. I was able to start processing what being alone was like and Gary was able to settle into new surroundings without constantly requesting that he be let out of his cage and sent home. He adapted to his new routine, the people and started to enjoy to the best of his ability being cared for, when he was always so used to being able to do everything for himself or having me to help him.

Time went by and I had to start working from home in mid-March as all government facilities were put on telework. The transition to working from home had its moments, with the hardest being all alone day and night in the house that Gary no longer occupied with me. It was depressing, exhilarating, fascinating and even though I knew I would be fine, because I was just surviving another period of trial and testing, it was a relief not having to see Gary in his transitioning state. I was grieving for the loss of the husband I knew and struggling with the acceptance of what was happening to him. I felt his pain, frustration and fright as I too was feeling those things. This time apart helped to give me time to decide how I could be at peace (as much as possible) with this new world. I prayed for everything and found myself being used by God to help others that could not find or pay for basic food items due to layoffs and shortages. I was able to provide for others, so I knew God was going to provide what Gary and I needed as we moved forward.

After four months procedures were being put in place that allowed for visitation. What a relief. Gary had time to mend from his operation and his terrible experiences with the skilled nursing facility, so even though he could not come home, he was able to walk well, tell jokes and laugh. His childlike nature seemed to be beaming from him in a different way and we were able to enjoy simpler things. He loved to have his hair cut into a Mohawk and on the Holidays, he wanted to have special bows put in his hair to match the Holidays or wear special sunglasses. He embraced his childish nature - it was fun and we could laugh.

For several months I was able to take Gary out to the park with the lake and the turtles where he could use his rollator walker to get around. He really enjoyed that time and we could social distance easily. I could only take picnic lunches or go through drive throughs as all the restaurants were closed for sit down service, so we enjoyed eating in the car together. We found ways to enjoy our time, despite COVID 19.

As the Holidays drew nearer, Gary's mobility declined, and he was moved to a downstairs room. This also impacted on the ability for me to take him out as I could not manage him on my own, so we spent our quality time in his room. His mind was getting further away, and he started to be upset and angry at his declining capabilities. COVID 19 had a major uptake as the Holidays approached and once again the facilities were shut down for an unknown period of time. This was upsetting as the girls were going to be with me at Christmas and part of our plan was to be able to give Gary a really nice Christmas. As it happened, it was very cold on Christmas, the home was shut down and we ended up putting his presents on the porch while the caregivers retrieved them to give to Gary and we watched him and he us through his bedroom window. He was able to hear us through the window, and we did our best to have a great time together for about an hour until we were frozen and had to leave. It was a special gift to be able to still provide him with happiness, but it was sad as well, because we could not physically hold him and kiss him. It was during these times that you learn to be grateful for what you have and are able to do – he could have not been alive or at a facility that we could not see him through the window or in a place that would not have proper care. We had all the positives in an otherwise negative situation. Thank GOD! It was another four-month span of time before I could see him, but at least there were phone calls.

As time progressed Gary moved to a different nursing home with more extensive care capabilities as his physical capabilities declined. Once again, the facilities were shut down and I could not visit for almost two months. Overall, in a twenty-five-month period I could not reach out and touch Gary for ten months, and for a period of two months within that time could not even talk with him.

Find the grateful moments everyday regardless of what your situation is - everyday is a different challenge and story, so be flexible, pray and keep moving forward to get to the next day.

Chapter 10

ESCAPE

I looked out the window to watch the movements of the man dressed in jeans, boots and red jacket carrying his white helmet, prepare his motorcycle for his ride. He meticulously checked everything, packed his necessities into the baggage area of the BMW cycle, straddled the bike, put on his helmet, started the engine and zoomed off. He exuded confidence, testosterone and his slightly tilted smile and dark sunglasses made me smile that I was so blessed to have him in my life. I prayed for his safe return and thought to myself that he would rather die than not be able to ride. Being a spiritual man his only desires in life were to have food (he loved his food), shelter, ability to ride and to be part of a loving family. He loved this freedom and fresh air.

He had been riding motorcycles for over forty years and at one point owned twenty-two motorcycles at the same time. He loved trail biking, Motocross and long-distance riding, motorcycles were his passion. When his disease made it impossible for him to ride, it was no surprise that he became very frustrated with his situation. To this day I feel the forced confinement slowly killed him as much as the disease itself did. He would often comment on what was the point of living if this were all he had to look forward to – I could not argue with that knowing who he was at his core.

He wanted to be able to be free to go when and where he liked without being monitored like a young child. As he transitioned facilities and moved through different stages of recovery from surgery to debilitating physical and mental decline from the vascular dementia, the move to the memory care unit in the nursing home provided the most peace for the whole family.

He wanted to be healthy. He regretted his decision to have the surgery. Living for eighteen months doing what he loved would have been better than what he was enduring. He would often tell me, "I wish I had made a different choice." I never said I wish he did too, because I did not want to burden him with any guilt, he had enough self-inflicted regret. His need for freedom had him trying to escape from the skilled nursing facility and he actually made it out the doors twice, setting off alarms, and having to have an alarm put on his wheelchair that would trigger if he tried to walk or if the chair got in a certain distance from the exit doors – it was a very real problem. He was never a fan of group settings, so even though the assisted living facility was a perfect fit in many ways he felt claustrophobic as he had a minimal area to move around in. He even tried to escape from the assisted living facility when the care givers were distracted, but luckily, he did not get too far. They did not anticipate his ability to figure out the gate latch in the backyard or how quick and quiet he could be in getting out the front door. The memory care unit at the nursing home was a locked portion of the facility with pin access for entrance and exit. He still tried to piggy- back a couple of times and was unsuccessful. He would not have been out of the building only out of memory care. This made us less stressed.

In memory care he had a long corridor and other space to vroom vroom in his wheelchair and pretend he was riding his motorcycle. Still not the same, but it made him happier as he had more roaming space. This provided a sense of peace to him and me as I knew he could relive in his mind his favorite rides of his lifetime.

He did escape his confinement twenty-nine and a half months later.

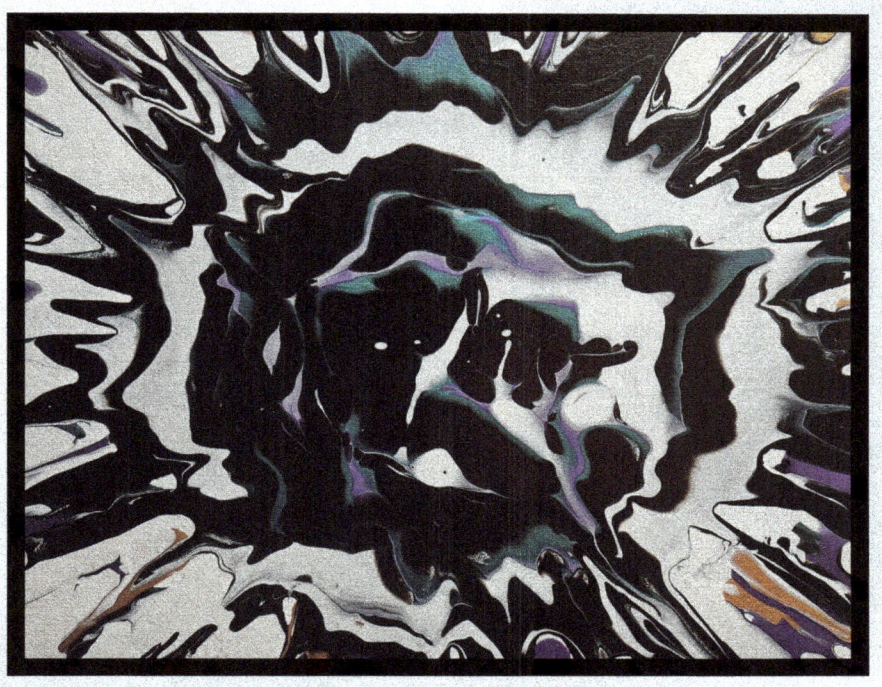

Two-sided Face

ECCLESIASTES 12:1 NKJV

Remember now your Creator in the days of your youth,
Before the difficult days come,
And the years draw near when you say,
"I have no pleasure in them".

Chapter 11

THE OTHER PERSPECTIVE

Looking up from bed I am wondering where I am. I do not think I am moving, but I have a sense that the world is spinning. Rats are running around me like they are circling their prey. Shivers and coldness cover me while struggling to move my legs to run away. Why won't they move? What is going on? Why can't I get away? Shaking is overtaking my body, and I am trying to scream, but it feels stuck in my throat. Where am I? Why is this happening? Scared, shaking and frustrated I realize I am trapped – HELP ME< HELP ME< HELP ME! Where is Linda ? Why isn't she helping me? I have to save her from the rats too – why can't I run? Blinking does not take the feeling and vision away. WHAT IS HAPPENING?! Why is this HAPPENING?! I should be able to run, I've always been able to run fast and not be afraid, what is HAPPENING? Feet are moving but not going anywhere – my hands are reaching out to fight off the rats, but they are not going away! Ouch, the pain, I feel myself shaking – they are starting to eat me! Arms rustling back and forth, grabbing, scratching at the rats, trying to pull them off me - not WORKING! Why God Why? What did I do to get eaten by rats? Screaming out "Help ME, the rats are eating ME! No one is responding to my calls for help – where am I and why am I alone?" I reach out and cannot find Linda next to me – where is she? She has always been there for me – where is she? "HELP, HELP, HELP MEEEE!" I feel wetness running down my face onto my pillow - I look at my hands and see red – what is this? Why are my tears red? The rats have gone away, I must have scared them when I started to pull them off my face and throw them across the room, thank God they are gone. I need to tell management that this hotel is not being professionally cleaned and maintained. I did not pay for rats to stay with me, let alone eat me for dinner. Do not know what all this red is, I have to get cleaned up, but I cannot get out of bed – Why? I used to be able to do all of this myself, what is happening to me? Moments pass, sleep resumes and then I hear "Gary, are you awake? Almost time for breakfast. OH my, what has happened here? You are bleeding all over your face – what happened?" I do not know, maybe it was the rats, what happened? "Gary, your face is all torn up like you were scratching yourself." "It had to have been the rats biting me", I replied. "You all really need to get the rat situation under control here. I cannot get any restful sleep."

When I arrived to visit later that morning, I found Gary all bandaged up on his hands and face. He was terribly upset and tired of being there, due to the perceived poor conditions and he wanted to leave, he was being overly aggressive and trying to get out of his wheelchair repeatedly to leave. I spoke to the nurses to ask: 1. Why no one heard him crying out for help during the night? 2. Why wasn't he given his Seroquel to help him sleep and to mitigate his nightmares? 3. Why wasn't I notified, so that I could have been prepared mentally before arriving for a visit?

The majority of the time it is important to go with the flow and not adjust a patient's thought process when they are not "with us" in our reality, however, there are times like this when, if they seem somewhat lucid, to try and level set their reality in an attempt to reduce anxiety associated with certain events/visions/thoughts. I explained to Gary that he was having a bad dream and because the disease made the dream feel so real he actually was scratching himself when he thought he was pulling rats off of him. He took this in and at least for a while seemed to help calm him down. Of course, the responses I received from the nurses went as follows: 1. Memory patients are generally awake a lot during the night and many of them go through struggles and staffing levels do not always allow for quick responses. I asked why there are no monitors at night in the rooms, but that requires special permission and authorization due to HIPPA and privacy issues. Understandable, but shouldn't safety come first for memory care patients? 2. I was told if they give him Seroquel regularly it could kill Gary. I responded with "you need to make him as comfortable and free of anxiety as possible." His doctor issued the script, give the medication to him. He is currently very upset, hasn't slept, which makes his situation harder for everyone as he is trying to escape, is mean and violent and can hurt himself or others. 3. The situation was managed and did not require medical attention from a doctor, so we did not reach out.

Keep in mind there are always policies, procedures, etc. to follow regardless of whether it is a government funded or private facility. Even though private facilities generally have higher caregiver to patient ratios than government funded facilities, there are still a lot of issues with getting quality care or a fully staffed level of care. Face it, any form of health care has major staffing shortages and memory care is not for the faint-hearted, so it can be even more difficult to attract people into that section of care.

Chapter 12

THEY ARE COMING TO GET ME – (RATS)

We all love to live in a fantasy land occasionally, but what if that state of delusion was with you most of the time? I do not think I would like it, so I cannot imagine that my husband did either. At the same time, it did take his mind off the fact that he was stuck in a facility for the rest of his life, so there is that.

Many times, I would come into the room and the topic of conversation would be how he was up most of the night trying to capture the rats. He would show me the paths they took and where they were hiding. The scary part was that he was all about capturing them and making sure that they would get killed. He would start talking about snapping their necks or stabbing them with scissors. Keep in mind that scissors were not allowed in the rooms, but Gary was exceptionally good at "acquiring" the scissors from the nurses when they came in to change his ileostomy bag. Point for everyone: the staff are so stretched that they either forget to take the scissors with them or they think they are hiding them in the room, so they do not have to remember them when they come in next time. Problem with that is when the shift changes more scissors are brought into the room. At one point I found four hidden pairs of scissors that Gary knew the exact location. Extremely dangerous for everyone.

To be clear the rat situation was all in his head, he was in a very good facility. The level of anxiety that he had due to his delusions was significant and some days he would laugh at their antics and others he would be very scared.

One day I came in to find him all covered in bandages on his face, head, hands and arms. When I asked what happened he said that the rats were attacking him all night and he had to fend them off as they were biting him. Apparently, he had been screaming and going nuts when the nurse came to his room.

This is where the rubber meets the road. I asked the all-important question " Is he on the Seroquel that the Doctor prescribed to keep him calm?" The answer I received was we are only giving that as needed when he is having a really bad time. I then asked so did you give him some when you found him as he is still very agitated and trying to leave his chair (at this point he could not walk on his own) and wants to leave. He is lashing out at me and my daughters. Their answer was 'no, because the use of Seroquel can kill him if we use it too often'. I said the man is dying already, can we at least try to give him some quality of life while he is still with us - give him the damn medicine or I will sue you!!!!

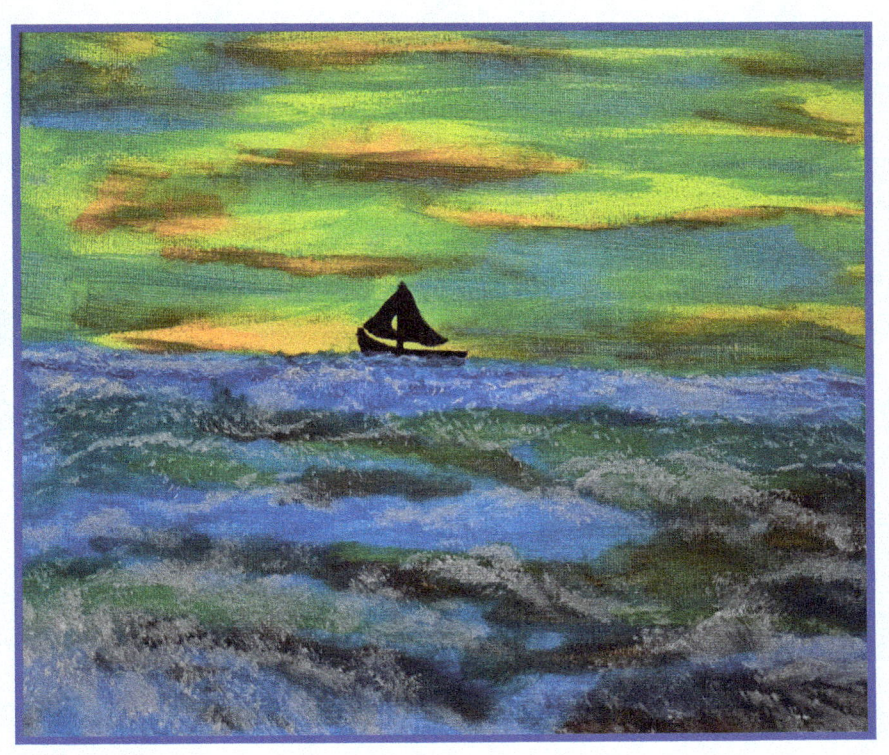

Churning Waters

Chapter 13

THE CALM BEFORE THE STORM

As I worked my mind was filled with the daily chaos of running a large directorate managing billions of dollars of funds on an annual basis. This chaos was my sanctuary from the personal chaos that had taken over my life. I kept the personal chaos covered by a mask while fully engaging in the organizational management that my training and career demanded. I have been a survivor all my life and this was just another level of surviving, so very few people outside my immediate family even knew what was happening in my life. I hid this very well with a mask of armor that was very rarely shattered. My armor was reinforced through continual prayer and as necessary crying to relieve the pressure of the emotions. My daughters and I became a source of each other's strength, and our bonds grew stronger daily throughout this journey.

Given that I still needed to work full time, and that Gary was heavy into sundowning by the time I would be getting done with work, I did not visit everyday – it would have been more than I could have handled. He was being cared for very well and it was so emotionally and physically draining that I could not have done both. As the days and months went by, I found that the best thing for both of us was to visit once a week. I decided Sunday was best, it was quieter at the facility and I had a day prior to recoup from the work week and prepare for the visit emotionally. There is no way to fully describe the level of emotions that I went through each week. As each weekend started to approach, I would start to feel anxious and upset. Part of wanted to be able to see Gary and the other part wanted to not visit. This may sound terrible, but the reality was that I never had any idea what version of my husband I would be encountering or what type of event may have, or be taking place, when I arrived. This was very daunting, scary and disheartening.

I remember sitting mindlessly in my chair trying to relax watching TV, reading or listening to music and my heartbeat would get faster, I would feel nauseous, and the tension just coursed through my body as Sunday grew nearer. Reality is that sometimes I could not bring myself to visit as his mind and body started to increasingly decline. To many of you this may seem heartless, but unless you have been or are going through this, you do not understand. Everyone has to choose what is best for them to survive this journey with a loved one. There are too many factors in each situation to apply a one size fits all approach. For those that may be reading this to support someone else dealing with their own or a loved one's journey – Do Not Judge or Tell Them How to Approach their Situation – it is important for everyone to be able to deal with their own needs in a way that will allow them to survive and not feel guilty. We put enough pressure on ourselves, we do not need others to add to the pressure - just provide love and support for whatever decisions are being made, unless specifically asked.

I cried and prayed before each visit, then put on a brave face and a smile to minimize any emotional response from my husband that would create an upsetting situation. Even with his mind going he could still read my emotions on several occasions when he was not with the Lumberjacks in the courtyard. Many times, after our visits I would sit in the car for a few minutes and just cry, because he would be in distress or having a bad episode or just exhausted and needed to nap while I was with him. There were other times I would cry and thank God, because we actually had a bit of fun, laughter and connection during the visit. He would sometimes ask me when I would enter the room – Oh you are back already, you were just here yesterday - it did not matter if a week went by, he never knew what day or time it was. His clock was measured by whether his stomach was growling and when the next meal would be ready – some things do not change (LOL). He did not even know which meal was when, just that he was hungry.

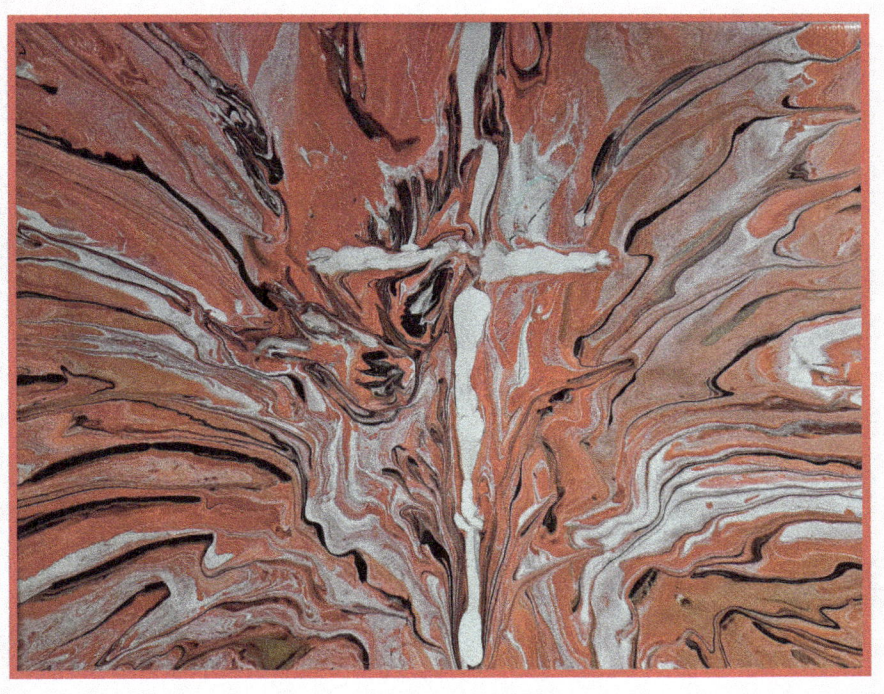

The Blood and The Cross

PSALM 30:10 NKJV

*"Hear, O LORD, and have mercy on me;
LORD, be my helper!"*

Chapter 14

HOW DO I GET OUT OF THIS?

(Fictional proposed account from the perspective of my husband, based on conversations with him)

The wind caresses my face as I fly by the familiar landmarks. There is a fresh scent in the air that smells of freedom and living free. As I take the curves there is a thrill that runs up and down my spine that cannot be described, I am living my passion. Forty plus years of pure excitement and relaxation like no other.

I open my eyes and see the never changing off white ceiling and light beige walls. No color except a few items hanging on the walls and whatever clothes I have to wear. I smell the odor of the hamper and trash can, no fresh air, except for what the two-inch opening from the windows allows to pass through my room. The view only changes with the seasons and I can imagine the feeling of being under the trees after riding to the park on my motorcycle. I remember trips from long ago that took me across various states and parks and randomly can recall teaching my wife and my daughter to ride, but those memories are getting further away and harder to reach.

I reach down and touch my legs to see if they are still there, because I want them to move and they aren't. Oh LORD! What is happening to me, why did I end up like this? I would have preferred to go out quickly in a motorcycle accident. I do not understand what or why this is happening to me. I hate being dependent on others as I have always been self-reliant and helped other people. Is this the test? To fully succumb to reliance on others? I am not sure I want to pass this test.

What will I do today and where will my mind take me when I cannot control it? I feel a float in the ocean, never knowing where I will end up or what will happen next. I miss the hobbies that I can no longer perform. I don't even know when or what people came into my room. My mind only minimally recognizes those that have been by my side for twenty-six years and even then, I cannot express myself appropriately, so they think I have no clue. This sucks. I DON'T want to do this anymore!

How can I end this? Do I want to end this? What impact will that have? GOD HELP ME! Please help me out of this situation and put an end to the suffering for all of us.

The bag is the key. Everything happened faster and worse because of this bag. I cannot even go to the bathroom like a man. I AM SICK OF THIS BAG! If I remove the bag everything will be alright, YES, that will make everything all right. It has come off by itself many times, but it was always able to be put back in place – why? What about that area allows the bag to be replaced? I have to think about that, not sure, I will have to watch more closely with what the nurses are doing and if I can, ask questions. YES, I need to observe and ask questions if my mind can stay focused at the right time. I will keep hiding scissors in case they are needed.

I believe several days have passed and I still want out of this situation. It is harder and harder for me to do anything on my own. I think I have the how figured out I just need to decide when I can do it. So much depends on my remembering what I need to do and having the physical capacity to achieve it at the same time I remember. This is definitely a challenge, but it is my last one and I am up for it.

Laying in bed, the nurse just left, this is the time. It came to me that the only way out is to really hurt myself in a way they cannot fix it. I am sure it will hurt but I have endured pain before and can again until it ends. I will use my fingers, that way none of the nurses will get in trouble from leaving scissors behind. I fumble until I find the bag and move my hand until I find where it attaches to my abdomen. I pull until I feel the moisture flow all over me and the sheets. I know this is not enough to do it. I reach into the hole and put my finger around what I feel and pull and pull - OMG – the PAIN! I start to moan, and I hope that this is enough to accomplish what I have set out to achieve.

I am in the hospital writhing in pain. The nurses at the home freaked out, that was an unfortunate part of this process. It also shocked most of the staff here at the hospital as well - I always have liked to be unique, and my death will be one for the books as well! The pain is a lot worse than I anticipated, but it makes me feel alive and for the first time in a while I have been able to accomplish something I wanted to do. I keep pulling the IV's out that the nurses put in and that is upsetting them, but I want the pain, until I am not in pain at all! I pray my wife and girls can understand – I know GOD will take care of them. I know I am on my way out and I have resolved it between myself, the LORD and my family. We have loved each other well and they have told me that I can let go. The pain was ending as hospice took over and injected me in my feet where I could not remove it. I feel my body relaxing.

I close my eyes and feel the air as I float away; I am on my motorcycle as I go from cloud to cloud and look down on passages of my life and think to myself - IT WAS A GREAT RIDE!!!

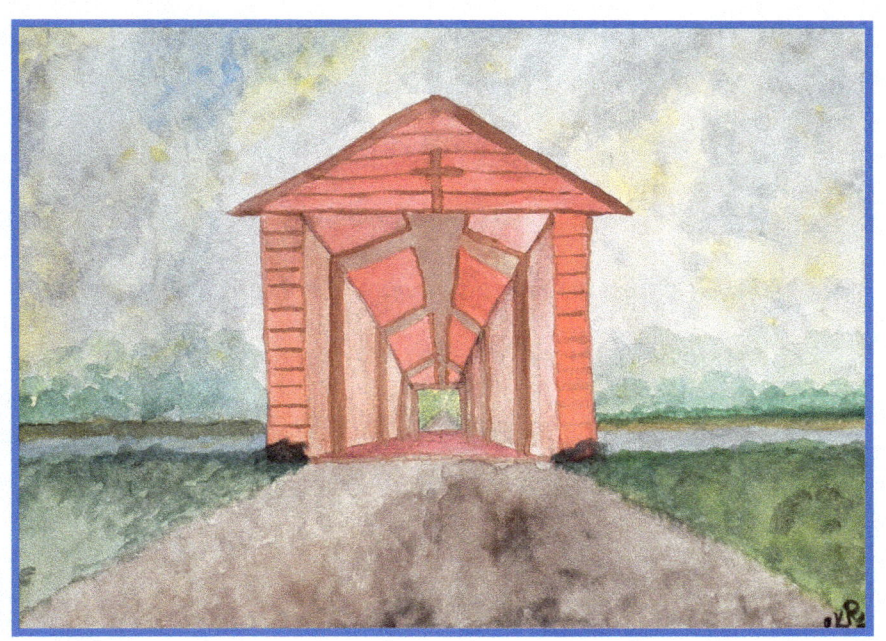

Crossover Bridge

REVELATION 21:4 NKJV

"And God will wipe away every tear from their eyes;
There shall be no more death, nor sorrow, nor crying.
There shall be no more pain, for the former things have
passed away."

Chapter 15

THE END OF THE WINDING ROAD

The call came around 8AM while I was sitting in my office at work finalizing my out-processing for retirement. It was my last on-site day at work and my official retirement date would be that Saturday. My sister and nephew were flying in to help celebrate the long-awaited retirement. It was to be an exciting couple of days to appreciate my career achievements and transition while embarking on a long overdue vacation.

I answered the call even though it came from an unknown number as I had a weird feeling come over me. It was an emergency room nurse at the hospital letting me know that my husband had been brought in during the night and that he was in a life-or-death situation that needed immediate decisions. My body and mind went into response mode, and I asked what was going on with him, "His bowel has been eviscerated and without surgery he will not live. I asked if the surgery would allow him to survive or if it was a hail Mary attempt to prolong his life. The nurse was not allowed to relay any types of odds or whether it made sense to do the surgery. I explained that Gary was not in any physical capacity to undergo surgery as if he even survived would leave him in worse condition than he was before this event. I demanded to speak to a doctor and to have them call me. I explained that I was at least an hour and a half from being at the hospital. Jackie called me after I hung up as she had received a call from the hospital as well and was already on her way down. I finished what I needed to do while awaiting the call from the doctor and as I just finished my out processing the Doctor called and I was told a completely different story than the ER nurse described. He told me that they may be able to push the intestine back in after shrinking it with sugar - I was like WTH! That did not make any sense, and I made him repeat himself as I explained that I was initially told it was life or death and would need surgery. A coworker was driving me as I did not feel that I would be in a good enough emotional state to drive myself and he heard all the back and forth and could not believe what he heard either. I became very frustrated and told them I would decide next steps when I arrived at the hospital. In reality, if it were truly something that could be remedied with surgery and would save a life under immediate need, they usually take action.

Jackie had received a call also and was already in route. When Jackie and I arrived at the hospital we were taken to his room, and I asked to see the Doctor. No one expects to see their loved one in a condition like I found my husband at the hospital. He was screaming in pain, and a nurse was holding his hand trying to calm him. I asked to see the problem and when she pulled back the sheet his bowel was distended from the ileostomy stoma - a lot of intestines were exposed. There was no way that they would be able to push them back in. The nurse knew he would not recover but could not officially say that. I spoke with Gary, and he knew that he was on his way to traveling the endless road on his motorcycle in Heaven. He just wanted to be out of pain and did not want surgery. They had been putting sugar on the wound as well, wound as well, in an effort to reduce the swelling and that process created a lot of pain. I knew at once that Gary was in his final hours. When the doctor came in, I got the same BS story that he told me over the phone. It was clear that he was a non-seasoned doctor who had no idea what he was talking about. He said that they were treating it and he could be sent home. I explained that the facility he was in was not equipped for this type of wound care.

In the meantime, the discharge associate came into the room and said they needed to send him back to the home as they could take care of him under their wound rehab guidelines. I asked who she talked to and what did the hospital tell them as there was no way this fell under condition for their hospice palliative care. I told them he was not going anywhere, and I called the Home and spoke to the head nurse. I asked her to come out to see for herself as I was sure that this was above their level of expertise. An appointment was set for 10am the following morning for the home to review his situation. In the meantime, I also demanded that the hospital needed to get the hospice/palliative wound care people to come see Gary. When we left, the nurses were trying to get his pain under control but in his struggles with dementia and pain he was pulling out his IV's. It was dreadful to watch and hear his screams. Based on the medical staff conversations we were told that he needed to be moved, so we left in search of a skilled nursing facility.

We received a call from the hospice/palliative care head nurse later that evening that they would be in to see Gary in the morning. We ensured that we arrived well before the time to meet with the nurses from the home and the hospital's hospice/palliative care personnel. Upon our arrival we discovered that Gary had been moved to another room. When we entered the room, a nurse was beside herself as she had been trying to give Gary pain medication, but all her attempts to provide pain medication were fruitless as Gary kept pulling the IV's out. By this time he had been in excruciating pain for over thirty hours while his body became filled with bacteria and started to shut down. We had brought a chocolate milk shake with us and Gary wanted some, the nurse said it wouldn't hurt him, so Jackie was able to help him enjoy a few sips of one of his favorite foods. The head nurse from the hospice unit came in and looked under the sheet and put it back down. As she did this the nurses from the home arrived and did the same thing. They said they could not care for Gary and they relayed that to the hospital staff and left. The Hospice nurse motioned for us to talk away from the bedside. She explained that she didn't understand what happened with his chart and placed a call for the ER department head to come up to the room. She was adamant that Gary was terminal and required immediate transition to end-of-life hospice care. This did not surprise Jackie or me, it just really created a whole set of emotions as we knew the day before in our hearts and Gary had now been in pain unnecessarily for over thirty hours. As soon as the department head examined my husband, she agreed that he should have been put into hospice upon his arrival. She had no explanation why the diagnosis on his chart was not accurate, but she was going to ensure that it would be addressed immediately with the attending physician. I immediately agreed to hospice taking over the care and they immediately injected medicine into his feet to mitigate the pain. Note: they cannot put pain meds in your feet unless you are eminently terminal and in hospice care, at least in Virginia at the time.

We had contacted Elizabeth a day prior when Gary was hospitalized and advised she should come up to see him, so she was already on her way. The hospice staff were not able to give us any idea of how long Gary had to live at that point, because they just took over and the dementia tremors could be confused with death tremors. They were awaiting blood tests for bacteria buildup to give a projected timeline. Gary was settling down into a peaceful sleep, so we said our goodbyes, told him it was okay to let go, and went to meet the family, have a meal and rest.

Gary went with the angels that night. He went fast, he knew we loved him, he was ready. We are haunted by not being with him at his passing and at the same time we believe he would have continued to hold on as he would not want to pass with us at his side.

The evisceration could have happened organically, as there are some statistics that once you have a stoma, sometimes the body just responds in a way over time to eject the intestines. He also could have accidentally pulled or caught the bag on something that created the problem, he never alluded to how it happened. I tend to believe that he might have intentionally done it, because he was tired of living.

There were mistakes made by the hospital that delayed Gary's ability to get the proper diagnosis and pain care he needed timely. I cannot get into details, however, all the issues combined created a perfect storm for a lawsuit. When we reached out to several different attorneys to determine if we had a case, they all said yes, but Gary's outcome would not have changed if the negligence had not occurred, so they could not foresee reaching a settlement that made it worth pursuing from their perspective. For us it was about accountability, so others did not suffer the same issues, but it always comes down to money these days, not about the suffering anyone endures. Be your own advocate for ensuring that you and those you love get the appropriate level of care.

There is no guarantee that you will not have issues when you advocate, but at least like us you know you did what you could do to try and prevent or prolong issues.

PHILIPPIANS 4:13 NKJV

I can do all things through Christ who strengthens me.

Chapter 16

LAYING TO REST

The call came in shortly after 3:28 AM on Saturday 30 April 2022 that Gary had passed. There was sleepiness, anxiety, numbness, sadness, regret and a feeling of relief that swept over me all at once. Everyone was woken up and told the news. Gary had passed quickly once hospice had taken over, he was farther along than they were able to determine, so there was no opportunity for them to reach out and have us be by him as he passed. My daughters, sister and I went to the hospital to formally identify the deceased. I have been to many funerals, but it is a different situation to have to identify someone who has just recently passed over and has not been moved from the place they died. The last time I had to do that was with my father forty-one years earlier.

The room was locked and sealed with tape with a hazmat area label on the door. We had to wear masks to enter the room after getting the nurse to unseal the room. The odor of decay was already in the air. What was once beautifully flesh colored skin was now a grayish color and lips were blue. His skin no longer had the warmth that made me feel safe, it was ice cold and stiff.

Yes, the overall features were of my husband, but the body no longer could be considered my husband as there was no laughter, no impish grin, no dancing green eyes, no soul, no movement. We all took a pause and then one by one went over and kissed him goodbye through our masks, made sure he was tucked in, ignored the bugs that had started to be around his wound and left the room.

There was minimal talking on our way back to the car after release paperwork was signed. As our path included making initial funeral arrangements the day before we were prepared with answers to where to send the body. I knew Gary wanted to be cremated, but other than that we had not set up any pre-paid funeral arrangements.

The next few hours were a blur. We returned home around 8am and breakfast was almost ready. My nephew, a particularly good chef, prepared us a really good breakfast feast to get us postured for the rest of the long day ahead. Our preparation the previous couple of days included looking up several different places that offered cremation services. We paid special attention to their overall appearance and vibe that was created as none of us wanted anything that was old-fashioned or stuffy, that was not who Gary was and it certainly did not fit us either. We finally found one that we wanted to go in person and that is where we had made preliminary arrangements the day before. We called to ask for a time to come in and finalize the arrangements. We were able to get in that day, so off we went and secured our funeral dates and service needs. The service would be exactly one week later.

It was also the very last day of the month, which meant that the memory care facility would be billing for another full month of care for May. We had to regroup and go the home to remove all of Gary's things so that we would not get billed. A lot of the things were donated to the facility or thrown out as they were worn out. The facility was very good about ensuring that we had minimal impact and a bit of grace if needed to get his stuff removed. Luckily, we didn't have to clean the room as well, just remove his things. One minute he was there and the next he wasn't – even the staff was very upset by his passing as he tried to always joke and have fun.

The next week my daughters and I spent a lot of time crying, reminiscing, sleeping, eating and preparing our eulogies and a photo array to play at the service. Even though it was a sad time in our lives this bonded us together in a way that we never anticipated. The Lord really works his magic when you do not expect it.

As the week went forward, we just wanted to be able to say our final words and have quiet time to process our grief. We made the trip to the crematory to say a private farewell and then we all pushed the button to move Gary's body to the next level of rest. We were then in a place with our private goodbyes completed, where we could proceed with the public service.

The day of the funeral tensions were heightened; there was chaos and battles as emotions were running high and everyone was exhausted. I was sitting in my room trying to unravel in my mind what I was going to say when a battle broke out due to feelings being hurt. Luckily after a few rough minutes with everyone not being their best, we were able to move forward and focus. No one joined Gary in heaven that morning, so the day accomplished what it was intended to do. It was a beautiful service; the girl's eulogies were beautiful and mine literally came together at the last minute.

The next few weeks were about recovery physically and mentally through a lot of sleep, quiet reflection, completing more paperwork and attempts to regain healthier eating habits that had gone by the wayside. Even though the grief process would be ongoing for a long time, it was important to be able to get up and live each day. This presented different for me as I also retired at the same time Gary passed, so I had no familiar routine to fall back on. I was in the midst of recovery, establishing a new baseline for my day and trying to focus forward on what possibilities lie ahead for me in retirement and without Gary by my side. I prayed a lot, cried a lot, slept a lot and read a lot. I was exhausted from years of being in survivor mode and working at a job that was extremely high stress. My mind and body needed rest. I was and am forever grateful that I was able to take as much time as needed to heal physically and mentally from the trauma, before having to embark on something new right away.

I used this time to start the cleansing process of going through Gary's things. He had a vast collection of motorcycle collectables and hand made motorcycle models, it literally filled our entire garage and a room in the house. This process took many different times and days as it would become mentally overwhelming. Most of his things were donated to thrift stores that help people with addictions, as it was too time consuming and brought up feelings of resentment that he did not take the time to cull the collection when he had a chance. This decluttering is finally done after 3 years post death. As each load went away there was always more to go through - some things got hung on to a little longer, because they caused an emotional attachment. Now I can say I only have a few things that truly make me smile when I look at them. I am continually going through my own things and really decluttering, reorganizing and ensuring things are in good order to prevent additional stress on my loved ones when I pass over.

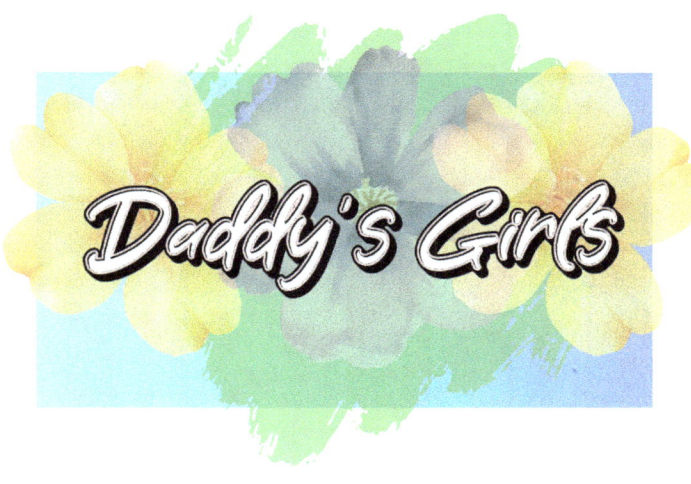

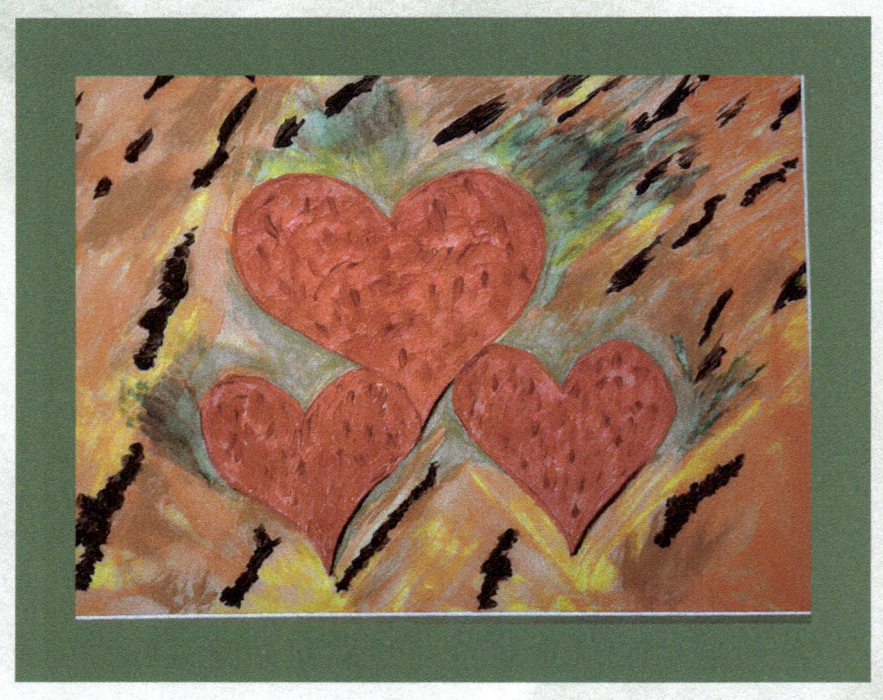

Three Hearts

Chapter 17

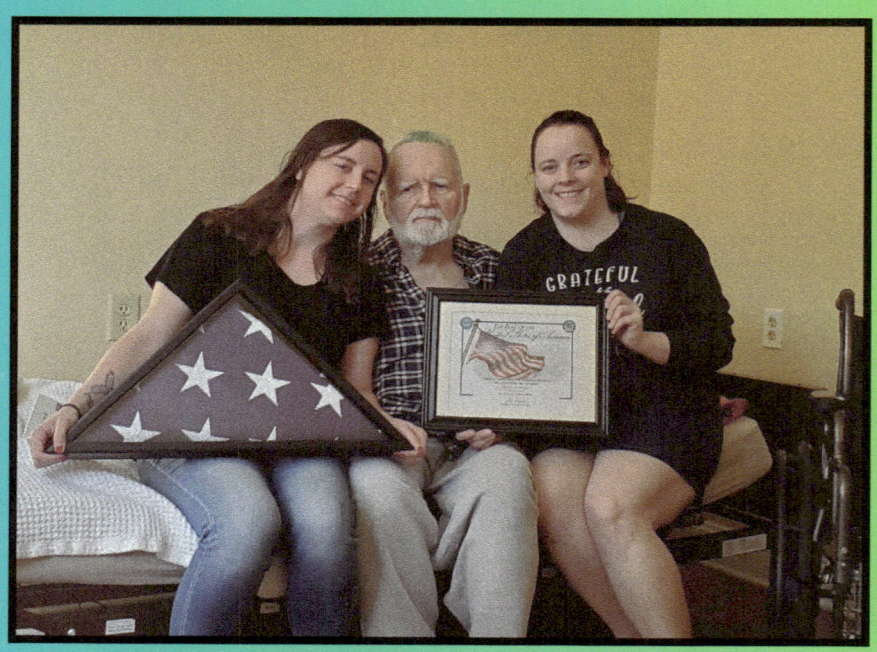

By Elizabeth Randall

A MIND UNRAVELING, A HEART BREAKING

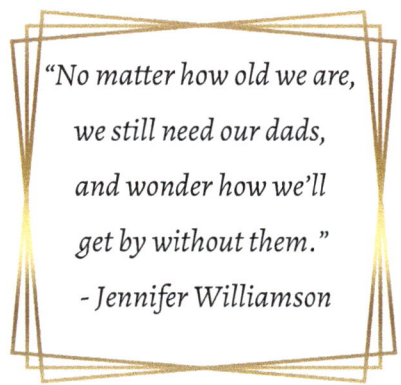

"No matter how old we are, we still need our dads, and wonder how we'll get by without them."
- Jennifer Williamson

If you've ever lost a parental figure, you know the profound emotional toll it takes on your family. When you lose a parent, there are often deep, raw feelings that seem to scream for attention—feelings that you desperately want someone to hear, so you don't feel alone in your pain, and so your grief can be acknowledged. Though the world knew Gary as my stepfather, he was my father in every sense that mattered. He raised me, taught me, and showed me what it meant to be loved unconditionally, not because of blood, but because of choice.

He wasn't the man who gave me life, but in every way that counted, he gave me something far more important: a sense of belonging. His presence shaped my world—his lessons, his laughter, and even his quiet strength. He was the one I turned to in moments of doubt, the one whose approval I sought, the one who stood as the steady figure in my life. He didn't need a title to be my father. His actions, his sacrifices, his love, made it clear that he had taken on that role with a dedication that transcended biology.

From the moment he was first diagnosed with cancer, through the relief of his recovery, and then the slow, inevitable decline brought on by progressive cognitive degeneration—dementia—our family was forced to face a painful truth: he would never be the same again, either physically or mentally. Though he was still the man we knew, the man we loved, the changes were undeniable. My mother had shared a life with him, built around routines and quiet moments, before dementia altered everything. Afterward, the house felt different—empty in a way that words couldn't capture. And when I returned home, the absence of his warm embrace, the comfort of his greeting, left a space that no one could fill. It was as if home had been redefined, and no matter how hard we tried, it never quite felt like home in the same way again.

Through research and conversations with medical experts, we learned about the effects of dementia on both the mind and body. We knew it was only a matter of time before Gary would lose his mental faculties completely and forget who we were. The thought of it was something I could never fully grasp—not because it wasn't real, but because it seemed impossible that someone could forget those they loved with all their heart and soul. It wasn't his choice, after all, but the result of his cognitive decline.

Thankfully, Gary held on to key memories. He never forgot who we were as a family. He always knew who I was, who Jackie—my sister—

was, and most importantly, he never lost sight of who my mother, Linda, was.

Much of the chaos and confusion surrounding Gary's diagnosis with small-cell carcinoma of the bladder was kept from my sister and me—shielded, I suppose, in an effort to protect us—until it could no longer be hidden. My parents realized they had to tell me the full story after an incident during a visit to see me in Brunswick made it clear that I needed to understand what Gary was going through. His long-term medical battle, including complications with his prostate, had reached a point where silence was no longer sustainable.

If Gary were standing over my shoulder right now, he'd probably ask me not to talk about this part of his life. But I feel compelled to, because learning the truth changed how I saw him. It allowed me to recognize the incredible strength it took to undergo treatment while still showing up for life—fully present, loving, and strong in all the ways that mattered. I moved to Brunswick in the spring of 2017, and my parents visited twice over the next eight months. It was during Christmas that year when everything came to light—following a moment I'll never forget. My mom and I were sitting in the car after a night out, refusing to go inside until one of our favorite songs finished playing on the radio. I didn't realize anything was wrong. But then Gary snapped. I saw a side of him I hadn't seen before…angry, frustrated, urgent. "When I tell you I have to go to the bathroom, I mean I have to go now," he shouted. At the time, I didn't understand the severity. Because I hesitated, we didn't make it inside in time. It became a moment that stripped him of dignity, though it remained private - confined to just my mother and me. He never held it against me; however, I've always regretted not reading the situation more compassionately. That night they told me everything. And though it hurt, it also opened my eyes to a deeper understanding of who Gary was and what he was enduring.

Over the next year, Gary underwent extensive medical treatment—chemotherapy—in a determined effort to rid his body of cancer. It was a grueling process. At first, there were no obvious signs of cognitive decline, and any subtle changes were easy to dismiss. He had always been a bit forgetful, occasionally misplacing things. But gradually, I began to notice small shifts—he no longer seemed to always have his pen, handkerchief, or flip-phone within reach. These were staples for him, part of his daily rhythm. He reminded me of myself during my rookie year at Norwich—always prepared to jot down a joke, directions, or whatever useful information came his way- because he had the essentials in his pocket. The flip-phone was mostly for receiving calls, though every now and then, he'd reach out to a friend or distant relative just to stay connected and in the loop.

One of the clearest changes came with his motorcycle rides. For years, weather permitting, he'd be out on the road every week. Riding brought him joy, peace, and a sense of freedom. But as time passed, those outings became less frequent. Eventually, he gave them up altogether. The strength and balance needed to manage his bikes, and even his own body, had started to slip away—and with them, a part of who he was.

If doctors had been more explicit about the emotional and physical toll chemotherapy takes on the body, I truly believe my stepfather would have chosen a different path—one that allowed him to spend his remaining time doing what he loved most: being with his wife and daughters, especially during the holidays when we came home to visit.

It was the summer of 2019 when Gary was first admitted to the hospital due to a cognitive-related episode. He was released a few days later after meeting the doctors' basic criteria for responsiveness—answering questions, however simple or seemingly unrelated they may have been. Just a few months later, in November, I got a call from my sister after a night out ballroom dancing. I had no idea that call would mark the moment everything changed. Life—and what I understood as "home"—was about to be turned upside down, and nothing would ever be quite the same again.

When I arrived to support my mother at the hospital after Gary's surgery for small cell carcinoma of the bladder, we thought the worst was behind us—he had beaten cancer. But the anesthesia left behind lasting consequences: confusion, memory loss, and emotional instability that would haunt him and all of us. Though his life had been spared, his ability to live it fully had not. The surgery had rendered him medically disabled—dependent on a urostomy bag, his cognitive functions diminished—and our lives were never the same.

For six weeks, I stayed by my mother's side, helping with medical paperwork and navigating the painful process of relocating Gary from hospital to nursing home, and eventually to a small group home assisted living facility near Richmond. Those weeks were some of the darkest in our family's life. We tried to keep functioning, but our strength often faltered. There were days when all we could do was cry in each other's arms, completely consumed by sorrow and exhaustion. Other times were spent arguing with staff, pleading for better care—because what Gary received at that first nursing facility was nothing short of horrifying.

What I witnessed there still shakes me. Neglect, disinterest, and cold indifference. Gary, in his fragile state, had wandered out of the building unnoticed, and it took over ten minutes to find him outside, alone in the freezing Virginia winter. The fact that someone in his condition was housed at the end of a hall near an exit door remains beyond comprehension.

I remember the guilt, the frustration, and the mounting tension within our family. The man we loved was physically with us, but mentally, he was drifting. Sometimes distant, sometimes volatile. He'd lash out unexpectedly, screaming obscenities that felt like daggers. And even though we knew it wasn't truly him speaking, it still cut deep.

A part of me still wonders if we failed him. Maybe we could've done more. Maybe we should've done more. But there's a truth I have to live with: none of us—my mom, my sister, or I—had the emotional or physical resources to become full-time caregivers. And knowing Gary, he would've never wanted to be the reason we gave up our lives. He wanted us to keep living, to be happy. In my heart, I knew two things to be true: I loved my work in Charleston, and if I stayed to become his caretaker, I would eventually grow resentful—not just of the situation, but of my mother. And that, too, would have broken Gary's heart.

This experience shifted our family's entire perspective on life. I picked up smoking again—something I hadn't done in years—after one night when Gary, in a rage, jumped out of bed and screamed at me like I was a stranger. Shaken, I left the facility at 1:00 AM, drove to a gas station, and lit up. By the time I got home, I'd smoked two. But later that night in the evening, on the cold back porch in Chesterfield, I looked at the stars and felt Gary's spirit whisper: "Don't do this because of me. I love you. I wouldn't want this for you." That was the last time I smoked. I threw the pack away and chose to fight forward—not through addiction, but through clarity and emotional healing.

Soon after, I had one of the hardest conversations of my life with my mother. I told her the truth—that I would support her and Gary, but from a distance. I wouldn't quit my job or abandon the life I had built. I hadn't made the same vows she did on her wedding day. It was brutally hard to say, but it forced us all to be honest about our limits. And in that honesty, we found a new closeness. My mom never blamed me, even if it hurt. If anything, it made us stronger—more open, more real.

When Gary finally moved to the small group home, we saw a difference. He received the attention and dignity he deserved. It was a small facility, with only 8 or 9 residents, run by compassionate staff who truly cared. After the holidays, I returned to work. I remember sitting in my car that first day back, overwhelmed with emotion, sobbing because I didn't know how to be "normal" again. But my coworkers welcomed me with nothing but compassion. They reminded me I wasn't alone—many had loved ones suffering from dementia, too. That camaraderie became a quiet source of strength. He stayed at this facility for about a year and a half before he eventually lost the ability to move around on his own. But while he was there, he was treated with dignity, respect, and real human care—something that had been missing before. That gave us some comfort. At least in that small home, surrounded by people who genuinely cared, he didn't have to feel forgotten or discarded.

Still, that period of time wrecked me emotionally. Depression hit me hard. I began grieving the life Gary would never get back, and the moments I knew we'd never share again. The nights around the dinner table where he'd sneak food off my plate just to mess with me because I was too slow. The laughter. The teasing.

I started thinking about the milestones he would likely miss. If I ever find my other half and get married, he probably won't be there to walk me down the aisle. He won't be able to play with his grandkids someday—won't bounce them on his knee like he did with my sister and me growing up, pretending to be a horse while we squealed with laughter. No more basketball in the driveway. No more surprise snowball fights.

The weight of those never-agains crushed me. It was more than just sadness—it was a deep sense of loss for a future that would now go unlived. My protector—my Gary—was slowly slipping away, and there wasn't a damn thing I could do to stop it.

To cope, I turned to alcohol. Weeknights, I drank at home until the buzz turned to numbness. On weekends, I started drinking during the day—sometimes until I passed out or made myself sick. I just wanted to shut it all off, to erase the ache for a few hours. But that spiral was dragging me into a place I knew I couldn't stay in forever.

My saving grace was Allie—one of my best friends and someone who never wavered. She was there during the darkest moments, like the time I collapsed on the floor of my apartment in tears, unable to move, speak, or breathe without choking on the thought that Gary wouldn't live to see any of the things I'd imagined us doing together. She sat with me through the worst of it. She reminded me that I wasn't alone, even when I felt like I was.

I never want to go back to that place again—mentally or emotionally. And I won't. I made it out, and I'll keep fighting to stay out.

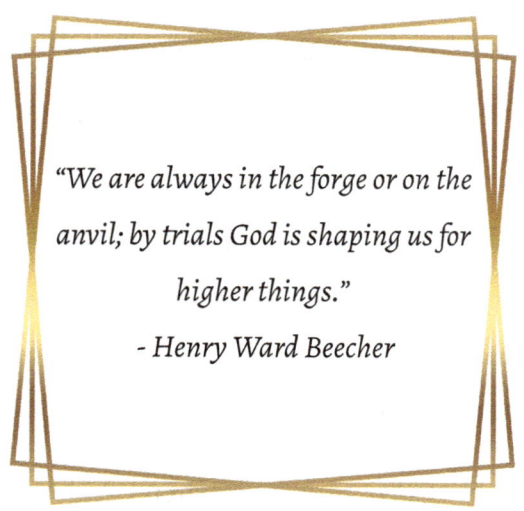

"We are always in the forge or on the anvil; by trials God is shaping us for higher things."
- Henry Ward Beecher

When Gary moved into the long-term care facility, it marked the beginning of the final stretch. His ability to move on his own had started to fail, and even the short bursts of mobility he had left soon disappeared. Confined to a wheelchair, his world became smaller—his days spent listening to music on the little radio my mother had bought him, and hours staring out the window at the tree line near the fence. He told us once that he imagined people hanging from the branches. It was haunting. Sometimes, he participated in arts and crafts, simple exercises we used to do as kids or joined in for movie nights. But with each visit, I saw the changes—his attention fading, his spirit dimming, his presence slowly slipping away.

I remember him telling us about the nightmares he was having. He swore rats crawled over him while he slept, that they ran across the floors at night. I truly believe that his past traumas—memories he never spoke of—were tangled now with his short-term recall, as the cognitive wires in his brain continued to fray and misfire. The neural connections were breaking down.

We did our best to redirect the conversations away from the darkness. We tried to ground him in better memories—reminding him of the "good ole days" and trading dad jokes, which had always been his favorite way to connect. Laughter had always been our way back to him, even if just for a few moments.

My last visit with Gary was in early March 2022. That was when we finally told him about the passing of his old neighbor—someone he'd known who had also struggled with serious medical issues. I watched his face as he processed the news, and something in his eyes changed. He looked down, then up again, and quietly said, "He was so much younger than me. Why am I still here?" In that moment, I knew something deep had shifted within him.

We tried to reassure him—that he was still here for a reason, that the Lord had a plan, and his purpose wasn't finished yet. Eventually, we steered the conversation toward lighter things. We even grabbed a balloon leftover from a recent celebration at the facility and started a spontaneous game of balloon toss. That brought genuine laughter—real smiles. Even Gary joined in, and for a little while, it felt like the weight had lifted.

But underneath the joy, I sensed we were all faking strength, even Gary. And when the fun came to an end, dread began to settle in my chest. If this was the last time I saw him, I remember thinking, at least it's a good one. One filled with laughter, not sorrow. Just under two months later, on April 29th, 2022, I got the call.

I was working from home when my mom and Jackie reached out. Their voices told me everything before their words even landed. I packed up what I needed and drove home. That night, after hours of updates and emotional exhaustion, we all tried to get some sleep. But I couldn't. I tossed and turned through the night, silently praying for Gary—asking the Lord to take him gently, to end his suffering.

It was nearly 4:00 A.M. when my mom and sister came into the room. "Gary's gone," they said softly. He had finally entered the gates of Heaven. His soul had been released from the pain and confusion he'd endured these last few years. Now, I like to believe he watches over us, reliving his life's happiest memories on a loop—surrounded by love and light, where the shadows of dementia no longer follow him.

It's been three years since he passed, and not a single day goes by that I don't miss him. I miss his bear hugs, the calm he brought to any room, and the way his optimism could brighten even the darkest moment.

> "The calendar whispers what time won't erase—a date still etched, a sacred place. I light a flame, let silence speak, feel his absence, strong and sleek. He shaped the heart of who I am—not gone, just far away."

Sometimes I find myself reminiscing about the quiet evenings we spent together—watching Bonanza or The Virginian. He loved those old Westerns, always sitting forward in his chair, humming along to the theme songs or quoting his favorite lines. And then there were the tickle battles—always started with that mischievous grin of his. He'd playfully tease us until we retaliated, and when we got the better of him, he'd stick out his tongue like a child who didn't get their way. It was never out of frustration—it was his way of keeping things light, making sure the house was full of laughter.

Those memories—the laughter, the playfulness, the light—are what I hold onto now. Because they remind me of who Gary really was, before the disease began to strip him away.

Author's Notes:

I would like to take a moment to express my deepest gratitude to the friends who stood by me during one of the most painful chapters of my life. Your unwavering support as I witnessed Gary's decline from dementia—and later, as I mourned his passing—meant more than words can fully convey.

Though not everyone is mentioned by name in these pages, please know that each of you has left an indelible mark on my heart. Whether you offered a shoulder to lean on, lent an ear when I needed to speak, or simply sat with me in silence, your kindness carried me through.

Your compassion and empathy have been a steady light during dark times, and I am endlessly grateful to have you in my life. Thank you for walking beside me as I continue this journey.

These individuals are my mother-Linda Randall, sister-Jacqueline Weathington (Randall), best friend forever-Allison Gutkes-Johnson, friends-Janet Hardwick, Robyn Carter, Kimberly Dawn, Brent Brodie, Robert McCune, Scott Bradley and Timothy Hall.

Chapter 18

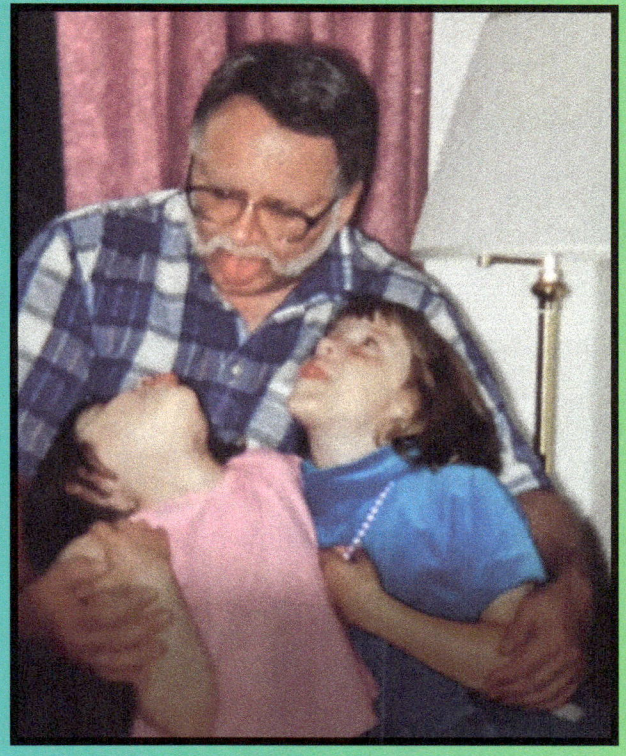

By Jacqueline A. (Randall) Weathington

UNRECOGNIZABLE

There I was, backpack slung over my shoulder, one hand on the silver doorknob when I turned around to say goodbye one last time. My mother holding him up, tears flowing down the sullen weak brittle version of the man I once knew. Standing with clothes hanging loose, unbalanced around him, violently heaving out tears, "I love you and will miss you," he said, as I walked out the door.

The image of him is haunting, the reality of the version of the strong caring alpha male that was my father... is gone, replaced by a man who lost all will, hope, and dignity in decisions of love to live longer, be present, falling away around him, around us all. I walk down the hallway of the rehab facility, out the exit into the cold frigid air, and yet it was crisp and free compared to the hell I left behind. I realized I could escape, but my father never would.

It's been three years since his passing, painful memories finally replaced by the good ones, childhood ice cream runs, motorcycle lessons, parallel parking, and the human jungle gym my sister and I would use him for growing up.

I got married last year, and as I walked down the aisle alone, I realized no one else could ever fill that place, it belonged to him. As I heard the music over the loudspeaker, and made my way into view, I felt him there with me, my heart burst as I knew he was all around. He was part of the blessing that gave me my husband, he was the light shining on our faces as the sun beamed into the church, he was present in the vows I made that life would separate us at some point, but I vowed to cherish the good and the bad until then.

In these three years I have cried myself to sleep, wept in a CVS easter aisle as I stared at the chocolate covered Russell Stover marshmallow easter bunnies that he loved, and I laughed, and smiled at the random moments and items that remind me of him.

Life continues to move forward, I am now pregnant with my first child. As I plugged the pregnancy announcement into my phone app to track a prospective due date, I felt your presence; the due date was my wedding anniversary, your birthday. I knew everything would be ok, that you were still here watching over us even though God had called you home.

I think of you in preparing the nursery, of the pictures of the family hanging on the wall, we think of you and praise you as we remind ourselves of our childhood traditions and the hopes and dreams, we wish to pass on.

Please note: Say "I love you" to your loved ones every day and never lose sight of the smallest moments. Do not let the world overwhelm you and pull you from what is important, the relationships we have with those we love.

Chapter 19

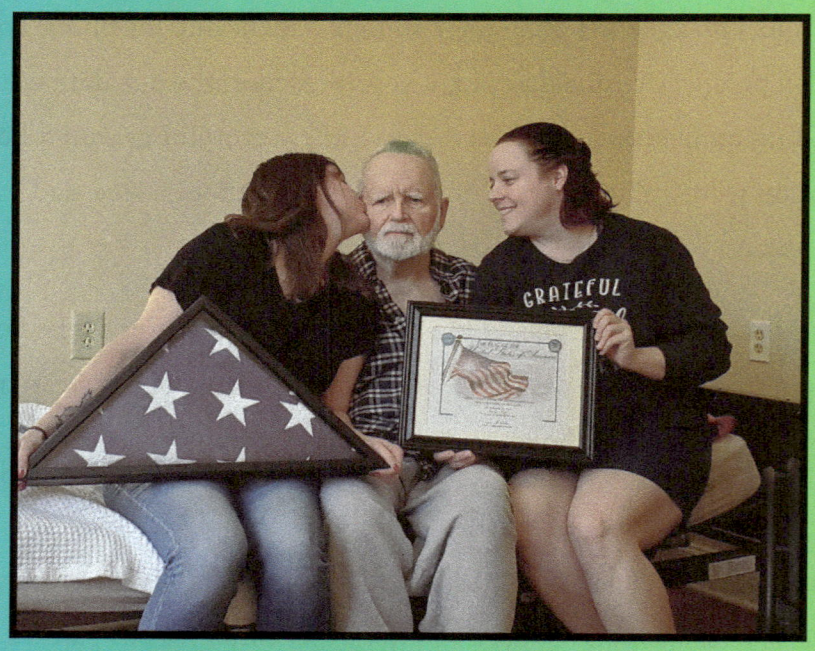

By Jacqueline A. (Randall) Weathington

EULOGY FOR MY FATHER

By Jacqueline A. (Randall) Weathington

This day is here, a day that my family has discussed, that we knew would come, and yet, it is still nothing like I imagined:

What do you say when you lose a loved one? How do you console a wife who lost the love of her life? How do you say goodbye to a father, a dad, someone you love?

The last two years have been the hardest of my life. There have been times I forgot how to smile, how to laugh, and how to live because it seemed I could only "survive."

I found this quote by Elan Mastai and I wanted to share it with you.

> "People talk about grief as emptiness, but it's not empty. It's full. Heavy. Not an absence to fill but a weight to pull. Your skin caught on hooks chained to rough boulders made of all the futures you thought you'd have."

As we come together today, and as I was trying to compose this message. First, I must talk about grief. The chapters of our lives cut too short, the futures we imagined, now, just hopes and crushed dreams. These last two years I watched a beautiful marriage transition from one of partnership to unimaginable sacrifice held together in the bond of true love. This sacrifice, dedication, and true meaning of "till death do you part" has left me broken, shaken, and without words. To watch as the life my parents shared now, a memory, and a house once filled with so much noise, (because Gary was very loud) now so silent.

We dealt with the loss of our father when he never came home from the hospital in 2019, to the holidays and birthdays he couldn't remember, to the times he was in front of us but not really there. Now we deal with the realization there are no more hugs and kisses, no more laughs and dad jokes, and there will never be a chance for him to walk us down the aisle or play with our children.

Now, enough of grief and the haunting thoughts of what will never be, let's transition to celebrate the undeniable force of who Gary was :

Gary was the greatest father a little girl could ever ask for . He has always been there and the memories we share prove that family is not defined by blood but by acts of love. My parents have shown me the true meaning of love, of partnership, and I cannot thank them enough for the example at which I hold myself and others too.

As I think of life without my daddy, it seems unreal, as though this is a joke he is playing but the punchline hasn't hit yet. Gary taught me so many things, there isn't enough time to list them all. As friends and family shared stories this week I was reminded of the many Pizza Hut buffet lunches we shared, the countless ice cream and goodie runs, and the little moments that never seemed so big but now inhabit most of my mind. Gary taught me how to ride a motorcycle, granted my first time out I crashed into the neighbor's bushes, but rest assured he was there to laugh and pick me up to try again.

Gary taught me that life cannot be fulfilled with "things" but that true happiness lies within ourselves and our relationships with others. Gary was his own man, no one and nothing could ever change who he was. He was kind, caring, hardworking, but he lived for the next adventure and made sure he listened to his heart.

When people ask if he is my dad the answer is always yes. He has always been in my life as far back as I can remember. In my heart I am still that little girl waiting at the top of the staircase for him to come home and play.

I have missed my dad for over two years; I have watched the life he loved pass him by and he couldn't be here to celebrate and live the life I know he loved.

I don't know what else to say except I miss my daddy, and I will hold onto the memories I have of him and remember I am still his little girl.

As we transition and say goodbye, I hope he knows how much I loved him, how much I've missed him, and how much he will be missed.

I know he is riding his motorcycle on the highways in heaven and waiting patiently until he sees his family again.

Thank You!

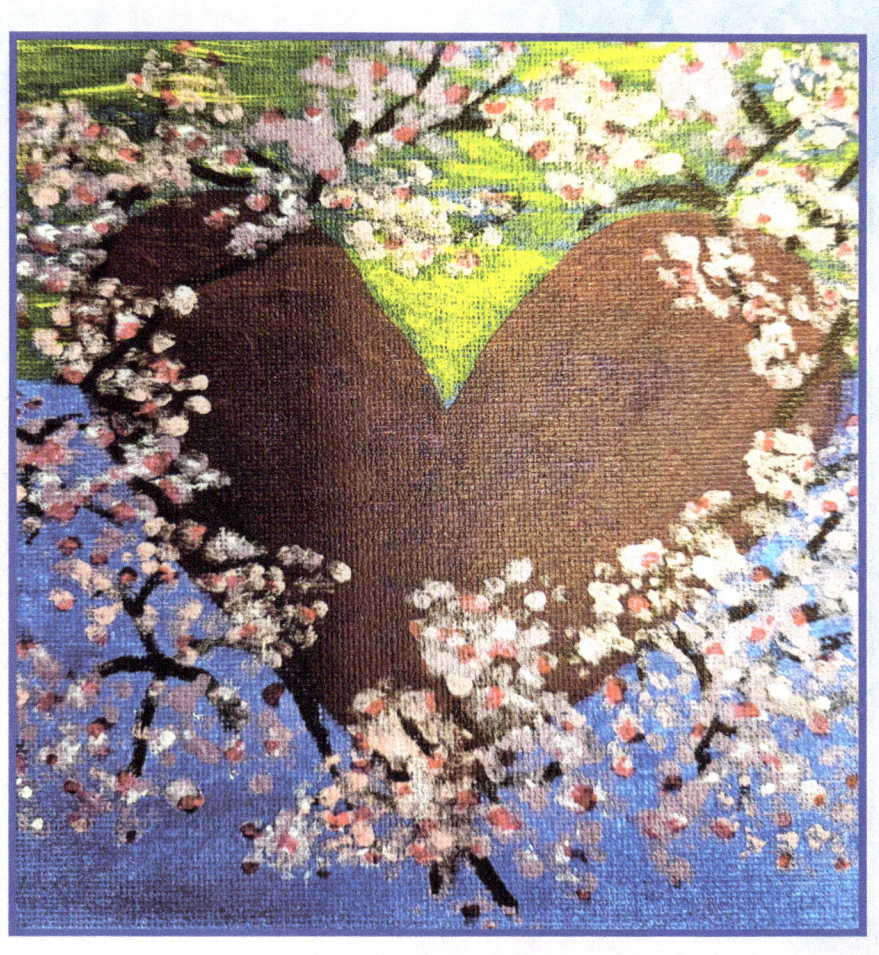

Heart

PSALMS 34:17-18 NKJV

The righteous cry out, and the LORD hears,

And delivers them out of all their troubles.

The LORD is near to those who have a broken heart,

And saves such as have a contrite spirit.

My Journal Entries

CANCER TREATMENTS

June 22, 2019

(Note: statistics are based on when events occurred)

A lot has happened since my last post. The health issues with Gary are very severe. He was diagnosed with an aggressive bladder cancer in early September that has a high recidivism rate. This particular cancer does have a standard treatment protocol with a good rate of success. We worked through the five months of that treatment plan fairly well. The plan included two bladder rescissions to remove tumors and weekly BCG (vaccine used to treat tuberculosis) injections into the bladder that were uncomfortable for Gary but were working to clear the cancer.

We were told in February 2019 that the cancer had gone into remission. Celebration time!! RELIEF!!! He still had two treatments to finish and then they would look into his bladder again as they had to continue to monitor for any signs of cancer.

We really enjoyed ourselves for two months and Gary's happiness was expressed by his appetite for all of his favorite foods; he gained fifteen pounds. Of course, this concerned me as he has to monitor weight gain to limit stress on his heart and not have a recurrence of the congestive heart failure that almost killed him in July of 2017. It was after that scare that we had a lot of really hard decisions couples put off and we had our wills, personal directives and Powers of Attorney put in place.

During the cancer treatments Gary and I became remarkably close and what it really means to love someone really hit home. We bonded in a way that couples can only do when they are faced with permanent loss of one another. It is a time filled with grief, love, happiness and empathy that really provides perspective to daily living.

On his follow-up, the ninth of May, another lesion (spot) was found on his bladder, so another rescission was scheduled. We, including the doctor, anticipated a recurrence of the cancer as we knew it was aggressive. Because of Gary's weight gain, and it had been over six months since the last visit, he could not have the procedure until his cardiologist signed off that his heart could endure the surgery.

His surgery was the fourth of June. The Doctor removed a two-centimeter specimen plus surrounding tissue while performing a complete exam of the entire bladder. The Doctor was surprised as he expected the same type of cancer recurrence, which would have been unusual based on the previous results, but the specimen looked unusual. We gave the Doctor permission to inject Germacticide (chemo) directly into Gary's bladder after he woke up from the surgery. We all knew this was not a good sign. It took Gary three days to bounce back from that outpatient surgery.

Our follow-up with the Doctor was on the thirteenth of June and that we received unbelievably bad news. The spot was an exceedingly rare small cell carcinoma in the bladder lining that represented less than a point sixty one percent (.61%) of all bladder cancers and metastasizes at an amazingly fast rate. This cancer is so rare there are only eight hundred cases known with only forty people documented in medical journals. There is no recognized treatment plan that has any impact on life expectancy. The median life expectancy for people at any stage of diagnosis is fourteen to nineteen months. Gary is considered stage 0. Recommended options to try and remove cancer and increase life expectancy include having a radical cystectomy (bladder, prostate and partial urethra removal) along with chemo and radiation therapy. Without those three treatments, life expectancy was between four to nine months. A ten-month difference with a lot of treatments and quality of life issues. What a shit show!

We have a three-day delay with our special oncologist due to a scheduling issue. That is probably a good thing as we have another weekend to "enjoy" not knowing everything - yes in this case that is good.

Gary is hanging in there, I believe he has been battling with his mortality issues since 2017, He seems to take most days one day at a time and appreciate what it brings. I have been really embracing the day-to-day approach as well, because other than items I really need to look at long term it is too difficult and sets me into an anxiety mode that is not productive or healthy. The whole family is impacted. On June nineteenth Elizabeth called me in the morning and that set off a trigger of events for the day. I feel her pain and needed to reassure her of her feelings so she could process and move forward. This then brought on a question from Gary whether I was doing o.k. and then he and I both broke down. We needed that – getting Gary to tears does not happen often, but we both needed a good cry! After an hour or so he was ready for some alone time, and I went off to work.

I worry about Jackie because she hates showing her emotions in front of me. I was tough like that at her age, so I get it – she does not want us to worry about her, but I do because I do not want her to break under pressure. I love them both so much it actually rips me apart when they are struggling with any problems – I know Gary feels the same.

So I sit here at what is now 6:17AM on a Saturday and don't know everything- as usual- and understand I am still processing – I am not ready to let go and I'm starting to analyze what roles Gary has played in my file – to say husband is easy, but it doesn't really quantify, as it means different things to different people. For me Gary has been the father to my children, my rock when things are tough, my emotional bouncing board, my lover, my friend, my confidant, my sense of humor and my entertainer. He has even been my guinea pig for new recipes, ideas, creative expression and overall career advice. He is everything to me and I cannot imagine not having him in my life. I hope I have been all of these things for him – Got to go cry now and hug Gary!

1 July 2019

This morning, I am feeling that it is getting very real, and I have been crying, and I am sad as we get ready to get the port put on Gary's chest. He will not ever look the same and I took a lot of extra time yesterday looking at his chest and enjoying it. I do not know if he will let me touch his chest after today.... It is like having a major part of our relationship possibly being torn away and it certainly will never look the same.

13 July 2019

Gary has completed his first round of chemo. He has to go through four rounds of chemo, and each round is 3 days a week every twenty-one days. The Doctor says he may have a forty percent survival rate of five years. Chemo, surgery then possibly radiation. Chemo was a very humbling experience. The first day of all the cycles will take all day. We met a couple of older couples and had some good conversations. In a different scenario we could see the possibility of making long-term friends. One of the husbands was on a palliative treatment plan to control the spread of cancer. It makes you feel blessed when you realize your cancer situation may be stabilized. I know forty percent does not seem like a lot, but it is better than what we originally thought. One day at a time. Three long days and the first round is completed.

25 July 2019

Well, it has been a long, tiring week. Monday when I came home from work Gary was out of his head. He greeted me in his underwear and two different pairs of shoes on the back deck. He was very disoriented and could not follow directions or conversations. He did not know if he had eaten or not or what he did during the day. I made a quick meal hoping his blood sugar was off as he did not have slurred speech, droopy facial expressions or other stroke symptoms. He was trying to eat dinner with a spoon out of an empty box before I gave him food. He ate little and he was so out of it I called my neighbor to help me get him dressed and take him to the hospital. Turns out he has an infection, and they have not determined the source as of today. There were no neurological issues, but the infection created a new heart issue that requires blood thinner, which cannot be done with Chemo. Lots of issues for the Doctors to figure out. Of course, the girls came home during this time and when we were not at the hospital it allowed for some major bonding time, heart to heart conversations, crying sessions and overall daughter, sister and mother therapy. We are going through a lot of thoughts to include not wanting Gary to suffer or to have a long-drawn-out illness. It is not good for any of us. We hope to be able to get a way forward so that we can work out the best way to plan the care process for the long haul. I need to get to bed -another early day tomorrow -

28 July 2019

This has been exhausting with the trips back and forth and in some cases twice during the day. Gary had an emotional meltdown Saturday that was long overdue and agreed to see a Chaplain. We held him and let him cry. He was distraught because he was told that he would be put in rehab and doing three hours of physical exercise a day and he did not think he would have the strength. He has been cooped up in a room under neoprene guidance as well as being relegated to either the chair or bed which were alarmed to warn the nurses of any attempts to get up. He is a high fall risk. His words " This is worse than being in prison." My heart breaks for him and I hope he is able to get some level of personal mobility so he can feel more like the man he truly is. His hair is coming out and that is adding to his anxiety as he loves his mohawk! I love this man with all my heart, and I hate that he cannot be the "whole" man he is at heart.

Trying extremely hard to take care of myself – it is not easy- we talked today about whether the dog should go with Elizabeth until Gary is done with treatments. He had been thinking about It already, so the discussion went better than expected. I am leaving it up to him. It is always tough when you have to choose between emotional support and health and safety concerns.

4 August 2019

Gary was moved to rehab this week, and he made great progress physically. At this point they feel he will make a good physical recovery from the infection; his cognitive and memory issues would still be impaired with no idea if any improvements might happen after Chemo is completed. His next round of Chemo is due to start Wednesday, but his ability to manage it will be determined when he arrives at Chemo and the Doctor evaluates him. Elizabeth left yesterday as she has to be back at work. She helped a lot with the house while she was here, and I think that is a form of therapy to help her deal with everything that is happening. I know she is upset because she will not be here when Gary comes home from the hospital, she loves him so much and has a lot of emotions running through her right now. I believe her distance from us is causing her a lot of anxiety. Jackie is here, so there is still support for when Gary is brought home. I am trying extremely hard to allow my emotions to just flow and not hold too much in but being careful not to create more stress. Not an easy situation. I have not had much alone time to process, but all of us are in the same situation. I have to be able to figure out how to manage his care with my ability to be on leave. This is going to be a long process and there is only so much leave, and the bills do not stop.

I hope Babe does not kick Gary out of bed as she has gotten used to his side of the bed! I expect Gary to crash into his chair as well as in the bed. He has not had much sleep over the last two weeks in the hospital.

13 August 2019

The week flew by. Gary was able to get his second round of chemo. We were on the go all day all week as we had an extra day of activity to get his Neulasta shot which will help with nausea and other side effects of the Chemo. He also had to be infused intravenously with fluids to prepare him for Chemo. I lost three of the eight pounds I gained due to the extra running around and preparing healthy home-made meals in an attempt to optimize our health during this journey. I always believe that behind every "darker event" are silver linings if we look for them. Gary is very tired and has finally accepted the use of the walker. I am able to do some work from home now, so that is helping with my stress level. I have realized that I have no real desire to work anymore, other than I enjoy some of the people. Retirement is looking ever more likely at the earliest opportunity, currently estimated at May 2022. I am going to try and be at the office most of next week – we will see – I worry about bringing germs back to Gary.

I am hanging in there and I had our neighbors over for dinner Sunday and I cooked up the catfish that they caught. We really enjoyed the fellowship, and it was a good distraction. I am getting into a good routine for all the chores, cooking, working and appointments, so it is starting to get less exhausting. I have Gary using a plastic urinal at night, so that he does not have to completely wake me up at night to go pee. I have been getting some of my personal health appointments taken care of to ensure that I am staying healthy.

18 August 2019

It has been nice the last few nights. Jackie came down on Thursday night and is spending time with us. She came with me for some tests I needed to complete, and we shared some good Mom and Daughter bonding time. She is struggling with a lot of issues, and I hope she makes choices that make her happy. She has the same kind of restlessness in her that I have had to struggle with most of my life – is there more? What if? It is hard to just "Be" without thinking about next steps or "What Ifs." Gary has really progressed the last two days. He loves it when she is here – he wanted to show off! I worry that he will not behave himself when I go back to work on Monday, but I have to have faith that he will do fine – I will only work a part of the day. He forced himself to the garage yesterday and then again to get the mail. He needs the exercise, but I do not want him to fall, so I made him promise to only do it if someone is with him. Hopefully, this will make him stronger, so that his next round of Chemo will be tolerated better. Jackie has planned to be here for his next round of treatments, and I hope to be able to get some personal time and go to work for a bit. She does not realize how much she is helping and worries she is not doing enough, but she is.

29 August 2019

Time flies! Gary finished his second day of chemo for this round. He is sleeping and the impacts of this week will really kick in next week. He is already experiencing chemo brain from this round. Overall, he has been doing good and has recovered greatly from the hospital stay. *I still take each day as it comes and ask the Lord for the strength to make it through the day.* I have been getting by, but some days are better than others. I have been able to work more and that is good and bad. I find I have more empathy for the people in some areas and then have no tolerance for other things that I consider basic responsibilities – I have really started to count down to retirement (1st date 9/11/21 or 5/07/22) could be longer, but not likely. Life is too short and as long as I can do it financially, I think I need to do it and enjoy not being on someone else's schedule. With the Lord's blessing hopefully Gary will be doing well, so we can do some stuff together. I have received positive results from all of my personal health testing and am incredibly grateful.

I have been really stressed the last few days as there have been a lot of things happening with the girls, I only pray the decisions they made make them happy and get them on the path they are destined to walk. I have considered going to a support group, but frankly not sure at this time when I would fit it in my schedule. I look to God for my help, but with all the anguish surrounding my daughters I cry a lot as I can only be their rock and sounding board. My biggest fear is losing my daughters in any way. The pain would be too much to manage.

Chemo yesterday was long, but we were able to engage in a fun conversation with two men next to us about funny old movies and it made the day go faster. It is weird that in a place where people are struggling to survive there can still be laughter and camaraderie – it is truly a unique experience!

1 September 2019

Well, the *"fun"* keeps coming. Last night Gary fell again. He was letting the dog out and did not take his cane or walker. He got dizzy and I could not hold him up long enough to get him to a chair. He landed in his basket of magazines and fell onto my grandmother's end table and broke a leg from it. He was a crumbled mess and thank goodness Jackie was here, because it took both of us to get him up. He did not hit his head, and the basket broke his fall. He said he was not hurt, but Jackie and I both strained our backs getting him up. This is getting really old that Gary refuses to acknowledge his need to require tools to assist him. I have to seriously consider admitting him to a home if he continues to not listen as I cannot deal with this every day. I had to be a hardass again and explain to him that it is not all about him and that he needs to respect what he needs to do in order for me and the doctors to help him. Then what does he do again this morning – goes into the bathroom without a can or walker and I had to rip him a new one – I am really starting to resent having to be a lecturer and hard ass – it is more stress than what is already an increasing level of crazy.

He almost fell again tonight, but he at least had his walker for stability. I was able to get him to a chair and tuck him in bed! LOVE - what we do for it and because of it!

14 September 2019

Time goes by so fast – the past two weeks have been challenging. I am struggling to keep up with everything – I am tired, frustrated and overall feel done in. My birthday sucked – no particular reason other than just counting down until retirement, no fun and spending the day in a dentist chair to get a crown prepped and a flu shot. Work has sucked lately and really only for the fact I do not want to be there with everything else going on. The people that know of my situation and management are being supportive, but I feel work gets in the way of me taking care of myself and my husband. I am exhausted to the point where I have issues sleeping. It sucked not being able to celebrate my birthday and it has been eighteen years now that I have not been able to properly celebrate as it has been clouded by events of 9/11. Whine, Whine – I know, whoa is me – get a life! Trying to have one – it just feels all topsy turvy right now!! We move into the last round of Chemo this coming week – we will see what happens next – should be surgery – who knows anymore -----

Gary fell again yesterday and has been getting weaker and dizzier as time goes on –

MRI on Monday – his second one – we will see –

22 September 2019

Gary has completed his last session of Chemo and now we have to get through tests and surgery. Lots of appointments the next few weeks before we get a date for surgery. He gets very weak when his blood pressure drops when he gets up – so he is back to using his walker – only with constant reminders from me. Trying to keep him from falling. I ordered a rollator walker so he can sit, and I can push him around if he is too weak to use it as a walker as his recovery from surgery will be long. His brain MRI came back normal, but I also found out that dementia does not show up on x-rays. I still believe most of the "other" issues are tied to exhaustion and chemo brain. Overall, a busy, exhausting week – we made it through. Gary did not ring the bell on his last day of Chemo – he would not tell me why.

I continue to try and focus today to keep it together. My patience is at its last legs and does impact my interactions with others, particularly at work – not good. Hopefully, since I am aware I will be able to adjust a bit. I just know I feel like work gets in the way of life as well and everything else! I really hope I have an opportunity to do some things I want to do without feeling "trapped" by obligations and responsibilities. Life is short – need to live it -------

13 October 2019

I realize a lot lately how incredibly boring my life has become. I never thought I would get to a place mentally where I did not have any more dreams, I thought I could actually accomplish. I have ideas, thoughts and things I want to do, but I am forever constrained by other responsibilities and no one that I can share some of these ideas with that can help me realize them. Gary has never been one to help with my dreams if there is no positive for him, other than to provide mental support. If it is something I can do that does not require any effort from him – no problem.

We are hoping to get Gary's surgery scheduled soon and with any luck he may be mobile by Thanksgiving. I am trying hard not to get in a negative place as we move towards the next phase of treatment. Gary has started to be more mobile now as he recovers from chemo, but the surgery will set him back for a while. The care aspect for post-surgery is unknown at this time, as the girls are low on leave, so I will not have them available and do not want to add to their already stressful situations. Focusing on getting through each day. I am sure Gary is hoping the girls will be here for his birthday in case the surgery does not go well. There is no indication of a problem, but it will be a long surgery and Gary's heart is not the greatest. I do not know if either of them can make it - feeling scared, sad and lonely –

9 November 2019

The last month Gary has been doing so much better that I have been able to be back at work on a regular basis. I am more tired between working and doing everything else. I have had to resort to some fast meals, but it is putting some weight back on Gary, so he is better postured for the surgery, but it is not good for my health. Surgery has been scheduled for the 20th of November, and I have been coordinating my leave between then and the beginning of January. I had to find someone willing to take on the extra duties for that period of time.

I feel really strange, because I have not rushed off to join support groups and add more stuff to my schedule. I guess when I need help, I just ask for it now, which I could never do before and *I know the Lord is providing what I need based on what I can handle – I'm tired, but I am at peace most of the time.*

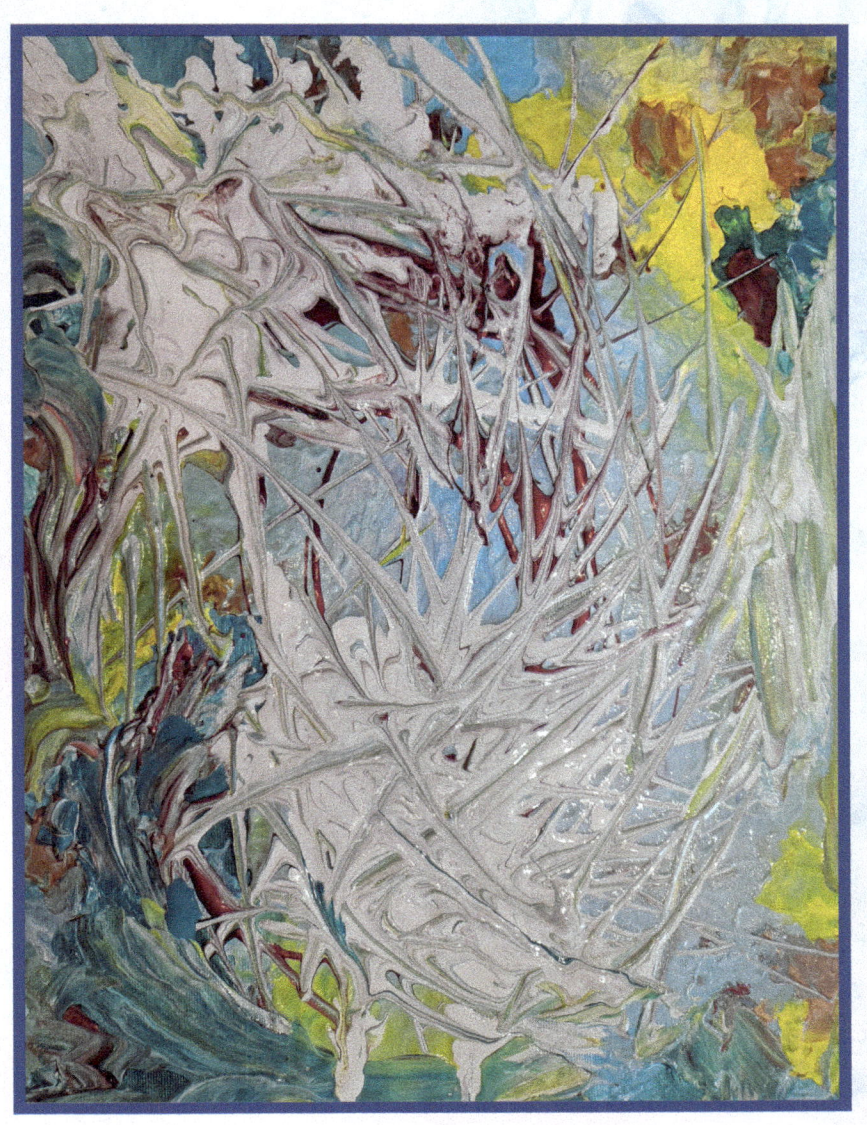

Delirium

POST SURGERY & DEMENTIA

(Post Surgery)

25 November 2019

    Hell is a good way to describe the last week. Gary's surgery was on the 20th. He had all the best doctors and they even discussed not giving Gary the additional anesthesia that they normally give patients due to his age and heart issues, but he had a major sensitivity to the medicine. He has been having an extremely hard time getting back mentally with us. He has been having a rough time not knowing what is going on and has had to be restrained. They had to call and have me come back in to calm him down as he does not know where he is or what has happened to him. His physical wound is starting to heal, but today he had diarrhea as well and they had to put him back on fluids. His blood pressure was extremely high, so they had to remove the IV on the weekend. Today the doctor is checking for intestinal infection. Personally, the care over the weekend was very subpar – the nurses did not know how to keep the ileostomy bag placed properly and it was a mess today and was leaking all over. The ostomy nurse had to change it right away and due to the urgency, I did not get my training on how to do it. Gary only had a few lucid moments today while I was there. It looks like a skilled nursing facility will be the next step as he is not well enough for regular rehab but is getting to where the hospital cannot do anything else to help him. He has to be out of restraints for twenty-four hours and calm before he can be moved. It has been hell and I cannot even write everything down, because I do not want to think about it.

It is taking a toll on the family and myself.

The doctor alluded today to how Gary needs to get stronger so that he can be strong for any continued cancer treatments – I am pretty sure that if Gary has to do anymore chemo, he will not do it – another case is the lack of quality of life worth the price of survival? The debate goes on – he is miserable now and is tired and frustrated – I feel the same – People want to help, but I don't know enough of the next steps to figure out what, when, who, where or why to get help yet – one day at a time, lots of prayer, lots of hugs and lots of forgiveness for those family members who don't want to engage with the issues –

I really hate seeing Gary this way and it breaks my heart; I Love him so and want him to be in control of his own wishes - --

8 December 2019

The last 13 days have been Hell – the LORD is preparing me for something – it will be interesting to see what that will be.

Gary was finally able to move to a skilled nursing facility on Friday afternoon – not really impressed, but at least he is not getting pumped with narcotics to keep him docile – like he was in the hospital. I am convinced that another week in the hospital would have killed him, because he would have given up. He lost 20 lbs. in the hospital! Very frail but getting his appetite back and getting more exercise. He is regaining his cognitive functions but still has sundowning issues.

Elizabeth came up the Monday after Thanksgiving after Jackie told her she needed to be here to help. We have been staying with Gary around the clock in shifts at the SNF because they are short staffed and really don't seem to have it together. I believe the staff is overwhelmed and work long shifts. That is a downfall of our for-profit Health Care System. The doctor is excellent and some of the nurses and aides, but many just do not care!

The last one and a half weeks in the hospital Gary went through a lot – testing, sitters, too many meds, no exercise – major staffing issues and there was noticeable discrimination among the staff – even Gary noticed and he was on another planet most of the time. I met some great people who stood out, so it is not all a doom and gloom story. Communication in the hospital and the skilled nursing facility is a major problem and impacts the level of care. I feel some of these issues have extended the period of stay and impacted recovery time. I cannot even imagine leaving him alone at the SNF as he has not been able to get timely help for any issues. We are able to keep him secure and eliminate fall risks, because he is impatient and would be trying to move about on his own and would fall and get his ileostomy chords caught on the wheelchair. He has already made a lot of progress, so hopefully that will continue – looking at options for care.

One day at a time – the doctor asked me today if I was a nurse, because of all the technical terms I relayed to him on Gary's condition – *I feel some kind of care or patient advocacy is in my future* – we will see ----

I am scared about any follow-ups with the surgeon and oncology, as Gary's luck is not that great – I truly believe from our discussion the last two days that he regrets going through with the surgery and chemotherapy he won't do again. This whole process has broken my heart and the girls have gone through hell as well – of course Gary has been very emotional lately as I think he has a hard time looking forward right now – Just being in the hospital and SNF is so depressing – praying all the time for strength for all of us --------------

19 January 2020

WOW – what hell we have been through. After 24/7 supervision of Gary in the SNF until the 19th of December, Liz, my sister and I are wiped out – what a "Fxxxxx" up mess- thankfully, GOD intervened, and we were able to get Gary into a small group assisted home on the 19th of December. Then came more paperwork, getting Uniform Assessments completed for Medicaid and Long-Term Care Insurance and financial considerations for the 90 days out of pocket expenses. I have notes as I feel I need to write something to help people and at the same time I want to forget the Hell.

There has been a continual flow of people here at the house for the last six weeks, finally got a week to myself before I go back to work on the 21st of January. I have been grieving Gary as he is no longer the man I married, and it has been killing me. The whole family is having a very rough time with this. I probably should have written daily; however, some things are better to not have in print.

Incredibly stressed, sad and will need to transition Gary again soon –

as his evaluation has him not being able to recognize anyone within 6 mos. and that was 3 weeks ago already. The paperwork process is a nightmare and is never ending. I am so done in and have no idea now how I will manage work, but one day at a time. Gary does not remember we lent Jackie his car for the last six months. He is recognizing me and the dog but really can't engage in conversation very well. So very sad – I love that man so much and this is not what he would have wanted – I think I am getting an ulcer – I have a doctor's visit in a few weeks again – Tums are my friend – I am tired of talking to people about this situation and I am struggling with residual anger of Gary not doing anything about his stuff like he said he would years ago. I have no idea what the next two years will bring, but I do know that currently I am considering changing my plans to retire.

I pray for all of our sakes that this process will not be years long. There will not be any treatments for any other physical maintenance for cancer, etc. as it is against Gary's wishes and it does not make sense to keep a body functioning when the mind is not. I have not included a lot of emotion in this entry as it has been all too much and during my continual emotional mess, I was not able – I am getting drained now --

12 March 2020

I cannot believe two months have gone by with no journaling. I have been getting back in the grove of work and coming home only to the dog. I am glad she is here. It has been a rough time, but I think I am finally at a place of resolve and starting to focus forward. Paperwork is still a big thing – still waiting on Medicaid's final decisions, so I have the paperwork from a financial perspective. I received that UAI a while back. LTC finally approved Gary with an effective date of 7 March 2020. This of course helps with my piece of mind.

The dog apparently is feeling the changes and decided to totally mess up the bed, my clothes and the rug in the bathroom – she must be bored while I am at work. Gary used to be with her all day. She knew she was naughty.

Jackie and I have started to sort through a lot of Gary's things. I was at a place that I was ready, and it helped Jackie learn more about Gary and process her grief. The whole grieving while he is still alive is a very strange real thing. The LORD made us extraordinarily resilient, so we will get through it. She was ready to see Gary. We had a nice visit with him – took him to the park that is near the home and then to KFC for lunch. He was happy to see her, and he did well, so it helped Jackie.

A global pandemic is happening, and it seems like the leaders of the world have all gone mad! Time will tell the overall impact on our lives.

Tomorrow is our 21st anniversary so I took the day off, because I am not sure what kind of emotions will present, and I don't want to break down at work. I am glad Gary is still enough with me to understand we have an anniversary, but last weekend he did not know when it was or how many years – incredibly sad. What is also disconcerting is that he and I both wonder if he is better off catching COVID19 to end his misery sooner. This seems harsh, but the idea of him walking aimlessly with wet pants in a nursing home and not knowing what is going on or who anyone is, is sad to think about. *GOD will do what is right for Gary and I so I do not dwell on it.*

I find that I have learned a lot about Gary while going through his things and bringing stuff to him to remember. This has helped me process and enjoy my time with him. I will always love him and he has been a terrific husband and father – the girls love him so very much!

I will be selling his motorcycle, scooter and his car soon – cannot leave them sitting around to rot and he would want someone to enjoy them. This whole process has profoundly changed me and made me more patient and aware of other people's needs – I believe I am a better person and manager because of it –

I have thought of many people that I have lost and getting older definitely takes faith, courage and stamina to want to continue, especially as those around you are taken – Live well, Live with Love and Laugh a lot!

(Life in asst facility and nursing home)
(COVID19, Brutal Killings, Protests & Riots, etc. not discussed below other than any direct impact to this publication, but it all added to the trauma)

21 March 2020

While it has been a while since I have journaled. I have not seen Gary since the 5th of March. All the assisted living and nursing homes are shut down due to COVID19. Since he is in a small group home, I am able to talk to him on the phone, so at least there is some communication. It looks like Gary will be approved for Medicaid pending the sale of his car and motorcycle and removing his name from the bank accounts. It is like erasing someone out of existence before they are really gone. I am still going to the office for work until all my employees have themselves set up for telework or are aware of the guidelines for continued appearance in the office. I am taking each day as it comes, because there is no way to predict what tomorrow will bring. The girls are safe working at their homes.

11 April 2020

What a month – a period in history that will forever change everything. I am working from home now and the homes are still on lockdown, so haven't been able to see Gary. I miss him very much. I call about every other day and he seems to be hanging in there, but for how long I do not know. Jackie and I have been making sure the home has supplies as sometimes they have had trouble getting what they need.

Given travel restrictions are also in place we are Blessed that we have permission to travel due to our government affiliations as necessity dictates. I know the likelihood of me being able to see Gary before he either does not remember me or if he gets the COVID19 is highly unlikely at his point – we are mandated lock down at least until 6 June. My love for my girls keeps me going. I love Gary as well, but I know that I have almost lost all of who he was already and have been mourning him for a long time now and have mentally prepared to lose him this year – even if it is not his physical body that is gone. I have to stay on top of his care now with all the paperwork and eventual transition to a nursing home. Medicaid has been approved – full coverage – shocked me!

Tears come and go for everything –

9 May 2020

I cannot believe another month has gone by already. For being home most of the time the days are going fast. Gary is hanging in there, but I do not have any real sense of how his decline is because conversation is limited due to lack of new things to talk about. I have been working on a healthier lifestyle. Trying to maintain a positive attitude as in reality this is a good test run of what my life will be like in retirement I do not get something else to do to replace working. It is becoming a period of self-discovery. Jackie and I have been able to bond with visits that allow only being together at the house. I have not cried much lately – I guess I am just out of tears and accepting my new normal.

3 June 2020

Gary is still stuck in the home with no visitor rights – I am thankful for our blessings every day, but the road is very bumpy –

22 June 2020

I found out that I will be able to schedule a visit to see Gary. Totally emotional over that – do not know when – can only manage so much stress!! Visits are very upsetting ----------

12 July 2020

Saw Gary last week – first time in 4 months – he lost a lot more weight – looks like a skeleton. He was able to retain and have a good conversation for about an hour – Good to see him, I needed that and I know he did too. I prepared for my visit my crying most of Friday and Saturday prior as I had been holding in a lot to keep sane – this is all surreal - pandemic getting worse –

24 July 2020

Jackie has spent the week with me. Teleworking during the day and enjoying each other's company at night. We have had two particularly good visits with Gary and today's trip was extra special. We took him on a short walk at the park, and we got to see a swarm of turtles in the lake – it was awesome and none of us had experienced that many turtles in a natural environment. At one point there were 17 altogether. We took him to Sonic for a meal and ice cream – he loved it – we brought the dog with us and that made him incredibly happy. It was a surprise so that made the visit even more fun – he was able to have really good conversation until around noon – then the sundowning started – I am thankful to be able to fill our time with good memories while we can.

I sold Gary's Yamaha TW200 this week – bittersweet – he loved that bike – glad to not have to worry about it anymore, but sad that a piece of Gary is not here – it was sad for Jackie too as he taught her to ride on that motorcycle, but she isn't in a place to care for or ride it now. Rearranged some furniture, so that the emptiness of Gary's chair was not glaring at me, making me sad.

2 August 2020

Elizabeth was able to come back up to visit and we have had some major bonding time. Our visits with Gary went very well – fun and good laughs – Gary was really happy to see hare and we ate well!!! Elizabeth was finally able to release some stress yesterday, because she was able to see him doing better than she expected and was able to make some more memories. She will come back in September and Jackie will come down as well, so I am hoping for a family photo of all of us as it has been nine years since our last one - too long!

3 September 2020

The last few weeks have been flying by. Work has kept me remarkably busy and then I have been visiting Gary on the weekends, so it makes for little down time. Visits have been rather good, but Gary is physically getting weaker – still stubborn as ever! We did a walk on the lake trail, but of course barely got him back to the car – had to hold him up while walking – he would not turn around when I wanted him too and kept moving down the trail. That is the last time he gets a walk without taking his rollator walker. We were supposed to stay in that day, but they couldn't readily find his walker. He promised to be good and listen to me, but that meant nothing. He pushes me and I am just going to have to push back – I strained some muscles getting him back to the car. We had a nice meal in the car under a tree. Spent part of the time going through one of his memory books and learned more about him.

Last night I did not sleep well, and I kept having weird dreams about Gary – not good ones – I believe I am mentally preparing for what will come next. I started to mentally write his obituary I will need to put it on paper and see if Gary approves. I am sure he would like input on what is published. Very weird – scary –

27 October 2020

Time is flying by ----Everyday blends into each other and I am always astounded by how quickly the day passes and I am once again tucking Babe into her spot on Gary's side of the bed. Jackie came down and we visited Gary on the Sunday before his birthday. He insisted that we come for the BD cupcake celebration on the following Monday evening. He barely knew who we were that night. That was the first time in ten months I had seen him at that time of day, and I cannot say it surprised me, but it did depress me, which is why I go early in the day.

The season is changing, and I have a gut feeling so much else will be changing again soon- it scares me even though I expect it. I am continually torn between wanting to see him more or to keep a steady routine to minimize impact on him. I feel like I am being roasted slowly over a fire pit while still alive -----

6 November 2020

I am visiting Gary again on Sunday this week, getting bored with options for things to do within his window of clarity. Last week I took him to the drive through dinosaur exhibit – we appreciated the change. I feel I should clean out the garage, but at the same time I am not really ready. He is still alive even though he will never be back here to see anything. It will be a year soon that he has not been home – hard to believe that much time has passed already. I still have my days where I cry or feel sad, but I have to say that I do not believe I am depressed – I am thankful for the positives in our lives and look forward to what life may have in store for me and the family. I am trying to take care of myself, etc. and would really love some sex – it has been so long --- Emotionally I don't think I could do that yet, because I love Gary and I would consider it cheating, even though he is no longer capable of acting as my husband. I believe he would sense a betrayal.

9 November 2020

Overall yesterday's visit with Gary was good. He is starting to have more random issues early in the day. He was fairly good with cognitive conversation; however, his coordination was considerably off and his visualization of movement of objects was at times 180 degrees off of what was really occurring. These types of issues had not been presenting themselves until right before our visits ended. Even though it factored in the time change the timing is still about 2 hours earlier than before. He is still stubborn and wants to be independent so that is good, however it can make for some challenging times during our visits as he wants and feels he should be' able to do everything he pleases. I cannot let him, of course, for both of our safety. He is definitely a person that needs to be watched. I will have to start being more mom than Wife – even more than I already am – I have to hold on to my memories to get through this --------------------

16 November 2020

Yesterday's visit with Gary was probably one of, if not thee, best visit I've had with him since his surgery last 20 November. He was really spot on mentally and even though he tires easily he did not have any visual or physical variances during our time together. We spent a bit more time together, because he was doing so well and the LORD provided a beautiful day for activity. We talked, hugged, cuddled on the bench at the park, kissed with our masks on and nestled his head on my chest – just like old times. Then we had a nice lighter lunch in the car and went back to the park and listened to some of his favorite music. I played "all of me" for him and we both reared up as we held hands. Then we listened to some cheerier music – good time. He was worried about his drivers' license as he realized that it would have expired and he said it was keeping him up at night – he was so happy to see that I had and had it with me so he could hold it. I am glad I did that – I knew his ID and a sense of self was especially important to him and the license was really hard for him to not have on him at all times. It made him incredibly happy. I asked if he wanted any of his Road and Rider magazines I found the other day to read and he said no, but not to get rid of them as he was "not giving up on my life yet" – he is a tough "Bo hunk" – he will keep fighting – I will cherish yesterday's visit as I don't know if I will ever have that level of engagement again during our time –

We of course still love each other very much and even though he may not be physically here – he is still with me all the time – he worries about me too and the house- he is amazing!

I realize this was a special day and I am not under delusions that our next visit will hit those levels – I just hope we can visit, COVID19 could put visits on hold again ---

20 November 2020

One year ago, today Gary went in for his surgery that forever changed our lives. I am forever thankful that the LORD brought two wonderful people into our lives to care for Gary on a personal level that was not possible at home or in a larger facility. It has brough some level of peace to the situation. Yesterday I was told that visits and outings would have to be stopped again due to the spike in COVID19 cases. We are able to do window and doorway visits, bring food, gifts and call. This makes me even more grateful for the wonderful visit we had last weekend. I am worried about how the news will impact Jackie as she was unable to be here for the visit last weekend as she originally intended. I know that not being able to hug Gary over the Holidays will really hurt her. Maybe we can hug in the doorway, but that would not make much sense. There is hope that by mid-January the residents will have vaccinations.

30 November 2020

Jackie made it down for the Holiday and we took Gary some green bean casserole and banana bread which he really enjoyed. We were confused when we arrived for our window visit and doorway food drop off to find another resident leaving the facility with relatives to go to a family outing. This prompted a major discussion on what the quarantine procedure would be for the person when they came back and also that it is unfair to the rest of the residents to subject to different rules. We wanted to take Gary to the park and not be around a bunch of people, but we did not come prepared for that as we were under the assumption there would be no outings, etc. It was a very distressing day. Anyway, when I talked to Gary the next day he seemed to be in good spirits and understood that everything was on lockdown.

8 December 2020

Jupiter is really close to the Earth right now and it will also be remarkably close to Saturn – especially on 21 December. The closest in 800 years and I can see it from my bedroom window between 430 to 630 in the morning – it has been beautiful to see – I hope on the 21st we have clear skies so I can see the merge of two planets – exciting.

There has been another new virus breakout in India that is trying to get contained - I think people need to just think about living for the day and not even plan for the future as the world is so unpredictable.

I really miss seeing Gary. The world affairs are really getting so out of whack I worry for the future of humankind. Everything has reinforced in me that I can survive on my own, but I need to interact with people on a regular basis, at least through the phone.

13 December 2020

Vaccinations will be issued to all residents in facilities. Mixed feelings on the whole vaccination process. I am tossed today whether to drive 40 minutes each way to see Gary for only 5 minutes from the doorway or just call – my heart aches! I feel it may be better that I do not let him be too excited by seeing me as he will want to leave the building and he cannot. This has been a long nightmare. The Holidays are coming up and he has been asking what we are going to do – who knows. He sounded depressed the other day when I called, not surprising – I would be and I am.

18 December 2020

Jackie helped decorate for Christmas. If I were going to be alone this Christmas, I believe that I would not have bothered to decorate. Thank the LORD I am not going to be alone. It is official that Christmas with Gary will be limited to a drop by with elbow bumps in doorway to pass off gifts/food. Very sad. He understands but it very much sucks. It will not be much longer until he gets vaccinated.

19 December 2020

Today Jackie and I went to do our drive by with Gary. We were able to visit him from the doorway. He wore a Santa hat and looked really cute. We were unable to get him some of his favorite food from the dinner we all liked, because it is closed down – so we brought him some Dairy Queen instead with a sundae. It was good to see him if only for a very brief encounter. He looks like he lost even more weight, but his spirits are good so that makes us happy. It was a good day.

21 December 2020

The winter solstice and the merging of Jupiter and Saturn to form the Star of Bethlehem, what an incredible sight that I was able to experience with both of my daughters! A once every 800-year event and we could see it with our naked eyes – praise the LORD! Another strain of the virus erupted in Europe and they are on lockdown again. I feel this is GOD's way of cleansing the human population and if we do not change our behavior nature will take us out. Everything happening is so very biblical. I still plan my retirement, but not sure what type of future is before us – I just trust in the LORD to provide a path – Staying Faithful and Positive!

25 December 2020

Merry Christmas – praise the LORD for keeping us well and sane through 2020. It is weird not having Gary here for Xmas – we will be doing a drive & drop by to him later, but will not be able to see him for more than five minutes and can't touch him – very weird times! It is good having the girls both here – time has flown this week and by Sunday night I will be alone again and probably will be for at least 3 weeks. We will see where 2021's journey will take all of us – it is getting scarier. Having very disturbing dreams ---- It ended up that we were able to open a window at the home and visit Gary (he had his winter coat on) even though it was an exceptionally cold day we stuck it out for a while. The home had taken pictures for the residents to give a gifts, so we got some really cute pictures of Gary.

31 December 2020

This past week has been great bonding time with the girls and we had fun and prayed a lot. I wish I could write that the New Year will bring major positive change, but it is only something GOD knows. All I can do is to continue to pray, be prudent and try to stay healthy and safe. Gary is o.k. so far and hopefully that continues.

11 January 2021

Gary seems to be hanging in there, but his memories of Christmas have already faded. I worry again that by the time I can really visit with him there will not be much Gary left – Stressful Times ----

14 January 2021

So much upheaval in our world and country. I feel changes in my emotions and how I want to live whatever is left of my life- trying to sort them all out. I feel that I am getting close to being ready to finish the removal of most of Gary's collection. Under the circumstances I will not be able to sell the entire collection, nor will I spend time trying to get small amounts of money for items or deal with a lot of hassle by dealing directly with people. I think the greater good is to donate the items so profits can help people – I have what I need, and I thank the LORD daily for our blessings, and others need whatever support they can get.

17 January 2021

I am getting bad vibes – I have the feeling something bad is about to happen – outside of the rest of the world crazy – I hope I am wrong. I think I need to take some personal days soon. I am at a crossroads for myself wanting to clear out more of Gary's stuff and refresh my surroundings. It is not an attempt to forget him, but I need to tackle the "elephants" in the rooms and the garage and make the spaces mine so I can be transitioning forward ----- He left me with a mess that for years I asked to be cleared out and frankly I am "pissed off" about it. I have no real choice but to give it away because the economy and safety and health concerns are not making options worthwhile. I don't feel I owe him anything at this point as far a finding a home for his stuff, because he didn't make sure it happened when he had the time and health to do so – he will never know anyway, and he never asks about his collection – I think he understands.

18 January 2021

Woke up with my path forward – I am drafting a book about Gary's and our journey. Started ad book note journal this morning – Excited -

19 January 2021

Jackie and I went to see Gary for a doorway visit yesterday – it was good, but he is looking scraggly as they have not been able to bring in a Barber for a while – I know he hates it when he is not groomed well. He is anxious to be able to escape for a while. We explained to him that he will not be able to leave for an outing until the end of February due to the timing of his projected vaccinations. He was not happy – "too long" he said – he specifically told me not to visit as it makes him more anxious because he cannot spend enough time with us. I guess he is spot on but we need to see him to keep him active in our minds, because we all are getting used to being on our own and isolated. It has been 2 months since visits were shut down again already.

25 January 2021

I was wrapped up in my own little world this weekend and I forgot to call Gary yesterday – that scares me – especially considering I spent three hours writing about us the night before – I feel like part of me is forgetting he is still alive. Isolation has taken its toll on our relationship – what pieces were left. I fear that I am moving on and will be slammed back to another adjustment period when visitation is reinstated. This is HELL for everyone in the family. One day at a time – Sweet Jesus!

27 January 2021

I am struggling with the decision to get the Moderna vaccine – I really want the natural one, but it is not ready and will not be for a while. Gary gets his vaccination this week. How can I take him out if I am not protected? There are more contagious versions out now – what a constant Sxxx Show – my ability to care is being taxed to the limit.

14 February 2021

Happy Valentine's Day to me. Another year alone, but yet I do not feel completely lonely. I know with all my heart that Gary loves me and I him – we will be until we are not. Last week he even said to me that he hoped I would have a great Valentines' Day and that he was sorry he could not get out to get me a card – what a sweet man! I will be calling him in a couple of hours – cannot see him as the roads are all icy from the first ever major ice storm in this area (at least since I 've been here) – I am tired of firsts---

25 February 2021

Got to see Gary Tuesday for his appointment and he has gained a few pounds and looks fairly good for his condition. He did rather well at the appointment. He has totally forgotten when our anniversary is so I reminded him it was coming up, do not know if he will remember in a few weeks. I need to send him a card, which will make him happy. Told today we may not be able to take him out on visits until April – have to double check on this, but the executive orders keep changing.

2 March 2021

When I was speaking with Gary on the phone the other day, he was not with it – it has been raining for the last three days and apparently that really impacts the brain processing for dementia patients. He wanted flags to put in his hair, because dying his hair would be too expensive. He is more downhill than any of us realize since we do not get to see him. Have to ask again about taking him out for visits. I am just taking life an hour at a time - ---

8 March 2021

If all goes well Jackie and I should be able to take Gary out this Sunday. It is scary as no one knows if the people vaccinated can carry the disease to others – I really question what the point is anymore. I have not been authorized to get the vaccine yet. Gary is depressed, hopefully it will pass.

13 March 2021

Happy Anniversary to me and Gary – 22 years married and 25 years together – what a ride. This is our second year in a row we are not together for it and he does not even know that it is our anniversary – it is sad. Weirdly I am accepting reality and am more anxious over the fact that we will be able to see him soon – Jackie and I are planning for next weekend. He technically is able to go out tomorrow, but with the time change tonight I do not want to take him out until his schedule is stabilized and I do not want to see him alone. Jackie and I are working thru too many emotions this weekend as well – I never know when something will trigger an issue so I want to be left alone this weekend.

18 March 2021

Well vaccine day is here – if something goes a miss I have had a great life and my message to my girls is to be true to themselves, live each day with greatness and give to others, if only through kindness – I love them both very much and I will always be with them. Please look after Gary and tell him I Loved Him with all my heart and soul and I will see him when the time comes.

22 March 2021

Saturday Jackie and I went to see Gary. We took him to the park and then to a Denny's for a nice leisurely lunch. He did well and we had some really good laughs and hugs! It was a particularly good visit. He was exhausted when we took him back – no surprise there – he had not been out except for on trip to the doctor in four months. He is still my Gary in many ways – he told Jackie "I have to sit next to my beautiful wife" – how sweet is that!

Cleared out some more of Gary's stuff while Jackie was here to help – so much stuff! All donated –

24 March 2021

Never a dull moment- had to admit Gary to the hospital on Monday as he had a fever of 101.9 and we suspected a UTI. Sure, enough it was and he is still there. Luckily, it was an early catch, so hopefully it will not impact his mobility severely. Yesterday he was already working with occupational therapy on his walking, and I told them to try stairs as well as he needs that at the home. They said that it will be done in rehab and that it will be a while. It may be getting to the time when I will have to look at a full nursing home with memory care. Needless to say, this is nothing short of a stressful trip to nightmare land. I was at the hospital over 6 hours Monday – did not go yesterday so they could stabilize him. I am going this morning for a while to see what is what, and I have to let them manage him – they were told his issues and were looking at sitters, etc. Jackie came back to provide emotional support and help with the dog. Very much appreciated – this is really wearing me out – I do not have much leave left, so I have to manage expectations. Gary was so out of it Monday I was really there for the doctors – not looking forward to today.

25 March 2021

What hell is this – yesterday I never made it to the hospital – a tire lost pressure as I turned onto the main road, and I had to deal with that – *luckily the LORD didn't have me get a flat and gave me the sense to turn around and to try and take care of it.* I ended up having to make an early appointment at the dealership to fix it, because the tire wheel key was missing from my car, so the two other places I tried could not help me. I also ended up really downpouring, so it was best I was not on the road as the hospital was clear across the city. I hope Gary does not feel I forgot about him. I tried getting an update from the hospital, but no one picked up. Exhausted and stressed.

27 March 2021

Saturday, Thank the LORD! What a week – Friday I used Jackie's car to see Gary. The day became a nightmare to a certain degree. Gary was able to get discharged. I was with him until about 11:15am and he was getting all set up for transportation back to the home. I had meetings I was to attend and he was still very delusional, but physically active. We chased worms, dogs and played a magic game with his hands clapping – incredibly sad and special at the same time. Anyway, they called multiple times regarding him being discharged and they did not get him on a transport until 4:15PM, then when they came, he pulled off his bag and it took another 2 hours before he actually left the hospital. Then I find out that the doctor called his script to the wrong pharmacy instead of giving a paper one to the Chief of the home to fill. They refused to call the doctor to have it redirected, so Jackie and I had to drive across town to pick it up, then across town again to deliver it to the home. What a day.

31 March 2021

I talked with Gary a couple of times this week and he seems to be really tired and sad. He probably cannot remember his previous stay at the home and is having to readjust. There is no end to people impacted with health issues from COVID19 and life in general. Two of the people who work for me are struggling to live right now – it is a lot for everyone.

Thinking of planning another sailing trip – I think I will go on my own – I need to start doing more fun things by myself and learn to live while I am alone. I am always with the LORD, so I am not lonely and I speak on the phone regularly, but I do not have many connections in this area.

2 April 2021

Have to meet Gary at the doctor's this morning for his follow-up. I will probably hold off going to see him this weekend as I have work being done on the house and he will likely still be tired. We will see – do not really want to struggle with him by myself if he gets hyperactive – sad ---

4 April 2021

He is risen! Going to enjoy the day – hope it is a quiet one. I will call Gary later as Easter is always hard for him as his mom passed on Easter Sunday. Gary is slipping away more and more. When I called today he thought is motorcycle charger was plugged in charging one of the batteries. He does not remember that they had to be sold. I did not remind him and simply told him that I unplugged the charger.
I think I should feel more upset that I am not running up to see him more often, but the pain of it is so intense that I cannot bear it – I do love him so very much and wish we could have had some retirement time together. I did get some good hugs and kisses on Friday from him and I hope that next weekend he will still remember me -----

11 April 2021

I had a very upsetting dream this morning. I was wading through piles of Gary's stuff decluttering and reorganizing when Gary came home and started to bring stuff back into the house and I started yelling at him and he started laughing at me with his little crooked grin. I realized how much I still loved him, but I resent his collection. I woke up and now I do not know if I can see him today even though I should because the dream was exceptionally real and the feelings are very real. I am angry and resent having to deal with his stuff, it weighs me down in a way I cannot fully describe but I feel like I cannot get to being me by myself while I am dealing with all his belongings. I am realizing that it is not just the collection but I am struggling with seeing him as a shell of the man he once was and yet I know he needs me. Who is there for me? I miss my spouse, and I miss what we will not be able to do together, and I feel stuck in quicksand with no branch to crab and pull myself out. I am torn between wanting to see him and having to manage him on my own – it SUCKS!!! I also worry that I will miss one of the few times left to be with each other where he knows who I am – we have been blessed he still does.

He is on another medication for a different infection so that makes me cautious about taking him on outings now – we will see ----

21 April 2021

I am down a rabbit hole that I cannot get out. I feel like I am so numb and lost even though I am functioning. I visited Gary on Sunday and it was an o.k. visit but I see him slowly drifting away – something has changed. Also, when we were getting ready to call his sister, she texted that she was on her way back to the hospital and could not talk to Gary - this made him terribly upset and sad – it broke my heart. He said that if he did not get to see her before she died it would break his heart. I reminded him that she had visited the previous year, and he does not remember any of it. I had him leave her a voice mail. She is in ICU again, so many hospitalizations. One of my employees is suffering from complications from COVID19 and will likely not recover - too much pain and suffering.

26 April 2021

Jackie and I had a nice visit with Gary today – we had a picnic in the gazebo in the backyard of the home and we had Babe with us so that made Gary happy. He got a bit ornery when it was time to leave because he wanted to get in the car with us and go somewhere. We cannot manage the dog and Gary on an outing – too much ---

6 May 2021

The week has been crazy with appointments for me, Gary and work. I was able to have a really good conversation with Gary on the days, so that was nice. Found out that my employee will be passing soon – I am numb, hard as stone and cry a lot at home. He was such a good person and worked well past when he could have retired. I am not going to do that – I want to do other things; this just reaffirms my decision to leave next year.

15 May 2021

I hope to see Gary today. It depends on how he feels. When I spoke with him yesterday, he was having tummy problems and did not know if he would feel up to it. Now that things are starting to return to pre-pandemic levels for activity, I am realizing how much I miss Gary and the little things we did together. I am sad and Gary is lost to me as the man he once was and my hart is still breaking – I love that man and I feel lost and empty while at the same time trapped because I cannot pick up and go somewhere for a few weeks to get away in case something happens.

25 May 2021

Life is a fickle bitch – one minute you are good and the next you are not so good. Work has been nuts. On a positive note, I had a wonderful visit with Gary and Jackie this past Saturday. We took Gary to the picnic area and to see the turtles. We had great laughs and Gary told interesting stories based on where his mind led him. He knows he can not remember well. When I asked him if he knew the name of the new woman that was staying at the home he commented " yeah, but I can't remember right now" – then he said none of us there can remember what we are trying to say and he snickered. We almost had him out too long as he was starting to get uncoordinated at the end of the visit. – overall good visit.

Jackie and I worked some more on decluttering – extremely hot – so only could do a couple of hours. I feel progress is being made; I want it done as I do not want to feel resentful for a long period of time.

My faith filled employee died yesterday, he is with the LORD now and out of pain – he suffered so much the last few months. This is hard on our workforce he has been there a long time and was genuinely loved.
I thank the LORD for all of my blessings – things can always be worse -
----

1 June 2021

Long week, celebration of life ceremony, visiting Gary and work – I feel like I am on a roller coaster ----

6 June 2021

The world is rejuvenating. I have seen a lot of deer, foxes and fireflies in my yard over the past week. It reminds me of how wonderful nature can be. Had another good visit this week and he enjoyed the deer videos I took.

Even though I am at peace with our situation I have been crying so much more, especially since my employee passed. I am appreciating all the little things because we never know when our number is up. I feel at peace and sad on and off as I try to make peace with my decisions for my next steps and mortality.

13 June 2021

I had a nice visit with Gary today. I took him new clothes and groomed his toenails and facial hair. This made him happy. He was able to speak with his sister today as well. I was happy to be with Gary today and I am looking forward to our time together, because I realize what gift it is. My employees' recent passing has changed something in me and is an example of how much we can impact other people's lives without realizing it. Live Life – Love, Laugh and Loosen UP!

24 June 2021

Took Gary to the primary on Tuesday and his bloodwork has come back with some issues. They have referred his results to the urologist and oncologist, so I expect I will have to be trekking all over again. Depending on outcomes there may have to be some other decision made regarding on going care. I have been in a wait and see mode and have been expecting a change. Gary really has not looked well since the UTI hospitalization and he is getting frail and weaker. THIS SUCKS! I have cried so much over the last 19 months I do not know if I have any more in me.

I found out today that another colleague I used to work with passed away suddenly at work. I REALLY do not want that to be my situation -

------

27 June 2021

My feelings that Gary will not be with us much longer are

intensifying and my gut is very rarely wrong. Last night at 10:43PM I was notified by the home that they moved Gary to a downstairs room. He is not walking well and overall does not feel good. When I spoke with him yesterday, he seemed very weak and tired. He also explained he was humiliated because he said "nursing students were watching him" when he was being bathed. Could be or he could be remembering something else - who knows. I have had to take an anxiety pill today, because I feel that I am going to have issues. The home was thinking of sending him to a SNF for therapy for mobility, but based on the lab tests I feel we are in a much different situation, but the doctors have not circled back. He will likely end up in the emergency room in order to figure out what is really happening – we will see how our discussion goes this morning. I am grateful for the time I have had with him. I hope he does not have to suffer a lot of pain. I think he is ready to let go, because he has seemed to have given up lately.

5 July 2021

I will be going to see Gary for the second time this weekend. They are having a BBQ this afternoon for the families. I had a good visit with Gary on Saturday, and he has adjusted to his downstairs room and likes it. His leg was getting swollen on Saturday and this morning when I called, he said it is not any better. I have a feeling when we take him to the doctor tomorrow, he will end up at the hospital, but who knows! I do not know if he did hurt his leg as his weird stories would suggest or if it is tied to a kidney issue. On Saturday he was in good spirits and does not appear to have any fear of being at the home, so I am reasonably certain it is not an injury. His conversations did suggest that he is getting tired and is not sure what else he can endure. I very briefly talked about the doctor and that it may mean some changes and decisions, but I think he understood the meaning behind my words.

At one point he asked "what else can I do for you" after he was successfully able to sign some paperwork. I quickly replied, "be there for me" and he said he did not know how much longer he would be able to do that. It made me sad and, on the way home, I cried. When I was speaking, I was in the context of that day's visit, but clearly, he is understanding his body is giving away. I wanted to let him know that it was o.k. to let go, but at the time I was processing his comment, and I could not bring myself to respond. I am not ready. I have to allow him and the Lord to guide me to make the right decisions. This is going to be a rough week I believe ------

Later in the afternoon he was pretty with it. He rushed himself a couple of times with the walker and almost fell twice, but we got him where he needed to be. The caregivers actually say he has been doing pretty well. His leg is not as swollen and he is putting more weight on it, so not real sure what is going on there – it was a nice BBQ, and we had fun. He has a urology appointment tomorrow.

7 July 2021

Well, we did not make it to the doctor today. The BBQ was way too late in the afternoon, and it created a problem with the residents as they were all in a "hangover" like stupor due to their dementia that morning, that made it exceedingly difficult to get them ready for the day. Gary apparently did not sleep at all during the night, and they could not get him to focus or move well to get him ready, and he was not mobile enough to go to the doctor. I was not happy and relayed that they should have realized that was a poor time to have the BBQ, especially when residents had appointments. This very negatively affects the availability of Gary into the doctor as they are booked solid. In wait and see mode always. On a positive note, Gary's leg appears to be healing, and he was relatively with it Saturday and Monday.

11 July 2021

My visit with Gary was distressing, he was not doing well today, physically or mentally. His leg was swollen again, and he was in the wheelchair. He was all over the place with his thoughts today and yet he was able to recognize his problems and kept asking me what was causing his problem and if it would get better. After a few times he said to himself – I have dementia. I explained to him that it was Alzheimer's cousin and that there was no cure yet. He said he was really bummed. It is so heartbreaking to see him struggle with what is happening to his mind and body. All I can do is let him know that he has no control over it and it is not his fault as he gets very self-conscious. He hinted on his embarrassment with others in the home due to hallucinations and bodily issues that he was concerned they were making fun of him. I doubt that is the case, but Gary has always been a self-assured and self-sufficient person, so having to rely on others for basic needs really upsets him. He is definitely going to be moved soon – I have to get on that this week as well as follow-up for the fourth time with the urology doctor about an appointment. I was advised by the home that sometimes it is best to take residents to the emergency room to get the ball rolling, as sometimes that is the only way to make something happen. We will see what tomorrow brings. Extremely rough visit. I think Gary is very confused and tired. He did not even want me to stay past two hours because I wouldn't take him to get ice-cream and see the turtles. He did not understand why I could not do this. I tried to explain that I cannot manage him by myself, and he really did not understand that. I feel extremely sad, and he cannot even see the dog because she is not allowed in the home. I am praying the Lord gives me the strength I need to do what I need to do. I have started to research and visit memory care nursing homes that are accepting new patients.

19 July 2021

Saturday's visit with Gary was good. He was with it for the most part and was able to use his walker. We talked and held hands – it was nice. I wore my red dress that I love and felt really good for a change.

26 July 2021

Friday morning, I woke up to being notified that Gary had been taken to the hospital with a possible stroke. *I had no idea what had really happened, and my first thought was to pray that it was his time to take him and not let him suffer anymore.* Then I started to cry – stress, being tired of one thing after another and not knowing. I called Jackie and she came down and we went to the hospital together. We knew it could not have been life threatening as the hospital did not call me directly. Gary was in the ICU on stroke watch, and he had been given TPA right away. MRIs did not show any indication of stroke. The doctor said that he likely had a minor or pre-stroke episode, and the medicine did exactly what it is designed to do and broke up any clusters. A battery of tests was done. Given it is the weekend, and he is still in the hospital, I am still waiting for some other results. Gary did not seem to have any issues from the event, and they are checking his leg and some other wounds and bruises that are not healing. There was no formal suggestion of abuse from the doctors as with his mobility and health issues these can happen in normal daily life and a fall resulting from him attempting to be mobile was most likely. This became the perfect time to transition him from the home to a full memory care unit in a nursing facility. I was able to find a really good private facility near our home that had one room available. Thank goodness for having Long Term Care Insurance. This place has an excellent ratio of nurses and CNAs to patients as well as a facility doctor that will be seeing Gary three times a week. The Lord truly has perfect timing.

2 August 2021

(Memory Care Unit in Nursing Home)

Last week was incredibly stressful and exceedingly long. After fighting with the case worker who truly did not understand her role and praying a lot for the Lord's help – I was able to get Gary moved to the nursing home. He is adapting well. He has been partaking in arts and crafts and likes his room and being able to have a long hallway to get to the meal area. He was feeling very claustrophobic at the home. I feel a new level of comfort with him at this new place. The Lord continues to provide and my faith is always getting deeper with everything that comes up. A lot of people came together to make it all happen.

8 August 2021

Jackie came up this weekend and we had a genuinely nice visit with Gary. He was like a little kid and demanded pizza, so we ordered pizza for delivery, and all ate together in one of the family rooms. Gary had been wanting his hair (mohawk cut) died green, so I brought some temporary hair wax and Jackie did his hair – it was awesome! He was so happy, and he was really chatty - many of his stories were really "out" there. It was a good visit, but he does seem to be losing mental ground at a fast pace. We are just enjoying our time with him because he is still a trip and fun to be around. Our love for him is without bounds. I hope Elizabeth is preparing for the major shift, so she is not all distraught when she sees him in September.

We worked on dismantling Gary's collection in the garage – lot of stuff taken to thrift store and old furniture that stuff was sitting on is staged to be hauled away. This process allows me to feel like I am accomplishing something, allows for grieving and also brings out feelings of anger and resentment despite the fact that our love is strong. Love, forgiveness, and acceptance for each other's passion made our marriage work.

Sadly, the collection is now a fraction of what it was, just like Gary is just a fraction of the man he was. It is still very heartbreaking, but I am at a point of true acceptance of the situation, and I know the Lord is with us, providing support for our path we need to follow. I will always love Gary but I am slowly learning to find myself and transition to my life without him by my side. I really do not like clutter and am working to really get to a place of only having things that make me happy and minimize the impact – could take a while.

13 August 2021

It has been a long week. Work is really draining me. I could not sleep well again last night. Part of it is that I still have a lot of anxiety when I prepare to see Gary. He was ordered to receive a chair alarm yesterday because he is trying to be mobile even though he is not physically able yet. He will be in physical therapy soon, hopefully it helps. I feel between work and what unfortunately sometimes feels like an obligation visit to see Gary, I do not have the mental rest I need to pursue my own interests. Gotta go visit –

It was a very nice long visit today. He wanted to snuggle so we cuddled on the bed. I reapplied his green on his mohawk, refilled his supplies and took him a sausage egg croissant. He had on someone else's slippers that were falling apart and I think they got swapped during therapy - the outflow of cash for replacing items, even though his name is on everything, gets expensive and no one pays attention.

Something really nice happened when I took my load of donations to the thrift store. I was worried that they would not want more motorcycle toys, but the really nice man was overly excited. He asked me if I was the same person who dropped off stuff last week and I said yes, he asked if it was part of a collection. I told him it was a collection that took over 40 years to develop. He said the process of me ensuring that his items were given a new home was a sign of a "beautiful love" and that he would pray for Gary and me. The guys love the stuff and made a special place in the store to display them with respect. This made me feel so much better about what was happening with his favorite things.

I finished decorating Gary's curio cabinet outside his door today. He does not even remember making some of the pieces unique. He is in his own reality the majority of the time now, even though he can still associate with us, but the times, places and why are confused. Love is what holds us together.

16 August 2021

I find myself migrating more and more to thoughts of retirement. I have been planning in my head the things I want to do. I am getting more & more anxious to be able to pursue these things since life is so incredibly short. My plan for many years was to retire this year.

Everything is confusing right now and I have to ensure the benefits outweigh any negatives. I have been aching to get to my writing and painting but cannot focus with all the energy drained out of me by work. Everyone says just "do it" but I have to be comfortable with my choice.

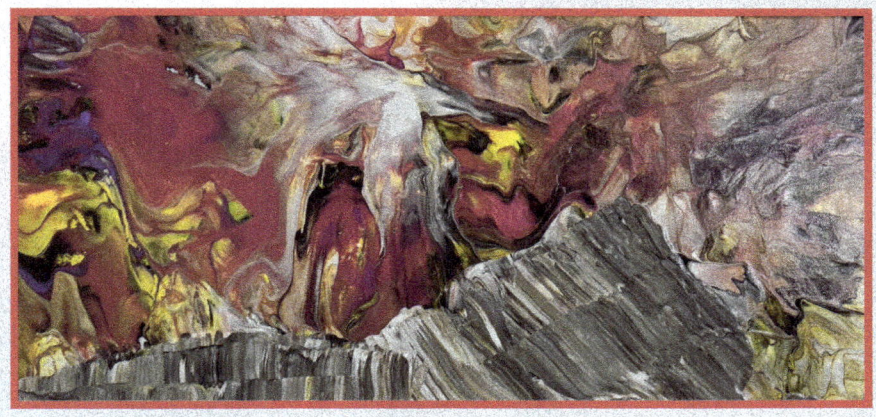

Chaos

DECLINE & CROSSOVER

18 August 2021

Today was yet another day in which the Lord guided me to a different path than what I thought the day would bring. I anticipated an early rise for an early start to the workday so I could leave early and visit Gary in the morning. The VPN network was down and it was an issue across that required on site assistance to fix. I decided right then to "opt out of work" that day. Instead, I rested, did some personal paperwork, visited Gary early in the day and took a much-needed nap. A person can only manage so much.

Gary was definitely glad to see me but his ability to know what day it is or partake in any normal conversations is degrading rapidly. He asked me today "how long will you be in town?" – not sure he really knows where he is past one hour of an event. His physical therapy is helping a bit to bring back muscle memory. I do not know if I should keep taking pictures with me to help jog his memory or not but I guess it cannot hurt.

He has taken to playing with his ileostomy bag again, so his room was really smelly today. Once they removed the laundry it was better but I ordered some odor killing gel jars and spray so I almost could not stay as it was so bad. I met a man today who comes to see his wife everyday and she is so far gone now that she roams around and enters other residents' rooms without any idea it is not hers. She has come into Gary's room numerous times and it really upsets him as she will make herself at home on his bed or chair and will not leave. Anyway, this woman still lights up when she sees her husband. Love does seem to be the biggest bond for the memory at least in some capacity ----

22 August 2021

My visit with Gary today was very weird! It gave me a wide range of emotions within two hours. Very exhausting - When I arrived, he did not realize I had come in because the door hit the back of his wheelchair. He was blocking the doorway because housekeeping was there. Once the cleaning was done, he was like - "how did you get in here?" – he did not remember me entering. He was all about wanting to see his sister before she died and she was only an hour away so he wanted me to take him – very demanding about it. When I explained that she lived over two thousand miles away in northern North Dakota he was like " What is she doing there? That is not where she lives---!" I was finally able to calm him down and we called her so he could talk to her. I do not know if she really understands his situation and I am concerned that she may actually believe him when he tells her about the mice and rats in his room.

After the call we talked a bit – memory joggers on trips we took and he relayed stories about the damn that is being built outside his window. He is concerned that it will block his view of the lumberjacks. It is always a fascinating journey these days. Then we were interrupted with more housekeeping and Gary starting his "I have to poop" marathon. Not a relaxing visit and he went from cranky to sweet and back to cranky again. He showed off his movements he can do, thanks to the physical therapy. If he really gets mobile again the staff will have their hands full trying to keep up with him.

The really special moment for me today was when he was ready to go to lunch and he said to me "I am completely head over heels in love with you!' – that made my day! Then we parted as he rolled himself to the other end of the hallway and he said, "see you next week." Gary never has missed a meal! He is a hoot ----

I am exhausted – nap time –

29 August 2021

My visit with Gary today was not real long as he is always on time for lunch! I trimmed his beard and brought him some things for his amusement. His main topics today were his annoyance with other residents coming into his room and waking him up or just making themselves at home in his bed. He said that one guy that came in and just peed all over his laundry – I believed that based on the mess I saw when I came in and the Director did say that all kinds of weird things happen in memory care.

10 September 2021

Time flies – I have been ill and trying to get well for Jackie's visit. Upcoming birthday and change in decades have been weighing on my mind. *I look back on my life thus far and realize that I have been Blessed. I have suffered various types of HELL but in the end those times allowed me to really appreciate the really important things in life - God always know best*

My emotional struggles the last few weeks lie in the realization that all my original plans for the future are now completely changing, and I am grieving the loss of those dreams while struggling to understand what my new dreams will be.

26 September 2021

After being able to get away for a while with Elizabeth we came back so she could see Gary before heading home. Jackie came down as well and we all went to see Gary. It was a very emotional day. He is slipping away at a quicker pace and he really was not with us at all yesterday. His conversations were all over the place and even though he knew who we were not sure he knew our names as he never used them. I could sense he was trying to bring the names to faces but could not either remember or could not vocalize them. He seemed depressed and he made a comment that he was still alive but that he was tired. Understandable given his circumstances. He also has someone in the room next to him that screams all day long "Help me I am scared" and most likely all night so I expect his sleep is severely impacted.

I feel that our time with him is slipping away. I just do not want him to suffer a lot of pain and angst during this final transition. I love him dearly and it pains all of us to see him this way and to only be able to "go with the flow."

Anyway, he was very distressed and had to tell me something but would only do so if the girls left the room. So, they did. He relayed some events that were really disturbing. Based on the specifics of the story and what I know of his background he was putting together multiple events of his past and the present for a new reality. He was terribly upset and asked for a large flashlight so he could defend himself. Of course, no flashlight was provided as given his military background and his determination he could have really hurt someone trying to help him or an innocent person that like him has no idea what reality they are in. This whole situation completely zapped me mentally and physically and it will be a while, if ever before I share this private moment with the girls.

The girls both have cried this weekend as they were really taken aback by his condition as they are not able to see him as frequently as I do. I still cry at random times or when a certain song triggers an emotion, but I am seriously dead emotionally at this point. That by itself disturbs me.

5 October 2021

My vacation has given me a different outlook. I am processing all my feelings in order to forge my path forward. For the first time I dreamed I was retired and doing whatever I want to do – I woke up revitalized. I also had a dream that Gary came home, and I was gluing his models together after they had fallen apart from age. Gary was walking but had no idea what I was doing or what his models were --- I awoke with the distinct feeling that it was time to go the final round with cleaning out his room in the house to include his collection of the models he made. After ensuring that the girls did not want anything I went to work and cleared out all but a dozen that were particularly significant.

Do not feel that I do not love Gary – I do – but I have to make myself happy. Gary is slipping further and further away, and I know that my future will not be with him. He still knows I am his safe person and that I am important to him, but I am not sure he knows why anymore. I do not cry much anymore unless specifically triggered by a song.

At our last visit a few days ago Gary tried to get me to take him to the park to see the turtles and when I told him he could not go because I cannot manage him by myself, he got pouty like a two-year-old and I had to hold my ground – played parent this time. He got over it pretty fast and then moved on to more stories about the Lumberjacks. He can still make me laugh but it is sad to see the shell of the strong man I married. *I pray that I do not succumb to this disease. It is really horrific! God has given me grace, patience and a sense of humor to get through this journey and I feel I gained these attributes because of it. I know the Lord is preparing me for my next chapter whatever that may be – I am calm and assured that everything will be o.k. It is with determination and strength of faith that I move forward* -----

16 October 2021

Time moves on, things change and my focus is all over the place. I have been cleaning out and doing minor updates to the house to keep me revitalized. Struggling with decisions to retire or wait. Visited Gary on Tuesday later in the day and was able to eat dinner with him and he was much more lucid for some reason – it was a really nice visit. Gary's birthday is approaching fast, and he has expressed that he wants pizza. Jackie plans to come and hopefully he will be with us during that visit. I continue to struggle with how often I can visit with my schedule, responsibilities and the emotional toll it takes on me. I do what is best for me to survive, at least once a week, sometimes more often.

31 October 2021

Gary's birthday, twelve days ago, was weird. He was all hysterical about rats biting him at night and needing mouse traps – it was crazy! He actually scratched himself so bad from the nightmares – he still has marks on his face. That visit was then followed up with a doctor visit the next day for his ultrasound and he could barely move from his wheel chair to the flat table to get his test completed. Nurses helped me getting him from the car but getting him back in the car was really a problem – he could not focus and the Lord sent me a strong man that I work with who was there for an appointment and just happened to be in the parking lot as we needed him to help. He helped Gary easily.

Today's visit with Gary was interesting. He wavered in and out of being present and it kept me on my toes! We called his sister, I hung some more pictures, cleaned his dresser drawers and closet and shaved his beard - we had a good visit. He was being a problem child as he got out of his wheelchair and walked along the bed (very poorly) and he said " I have to take risks if I am ever getting out of this place" – understand but he will likely fall and break a hip – I told him he was making me nervous and if he did not sit down I would leave – he settled down – he is such an anomaly! The doctor says his blood work and kidney function is fine - he may end up being one of those people that lives for ten years but does not know where he is – what a pitiful way to live. I am doing my best to enjoy the visit as like today we had fun – we played balloon toss with his birthday balloon – it was fun!

20 November 2021

The last few weeks have been remarkably busy, and I have been ill for at least two weeks. I have not been able to visit Gary because of being sick and the number of COVID cases are rising again. Still waiting for my booster. Made the decision to retire in the spring, getting everything in order prior to that. Hopefully, I can see Gary soon.

28 November 2021

The girls and I were able to see Gary for Thanksgiving and it was a good visit. Who knows what next year will bring but this year us girls will all be together at Christmas and hopefully we will have no issues visiting Gary. He is pretty much out of it, but he still knows all of us. He is in a world unto his own with his main fascination on getting his beard and hair done. He still has a good sense of humor but is not able to tell the jokes he wants to but will laugh when we tell them. The girls are always heartbroken after a visit, and it is making it harder and harder for them to visit. Visiting Gary is part of my life, and I must endure to catch a glimpse of the man I married. This is taking a huge toll on the family. This could still go on for a long time – God only knows.

14 December 2021

Processing a lot of personal issues and emotions. Spent some good time with Gary on Sunday and tidied him up so that it made him happy which in turn made me happy.

29 January 2022

I cannot believe I am getting to a place that I am not writing more often. The Holidays have come and gone. Enjoyed time with the girls and Gary. I committed to my retirement date and that has made more work at the office. Jackie and I have refurbished Gary's modeling room as an extra spare room. There was a four-week period that I could not visit Gary due to COVID shutdown at the facilities again. Could not even call him as he cannot have a phone and they cannot accommodate running around to bring residents to the phone. Time is passing quickly.

13 March 2022

The paperwork is submitted for a retirement date of 30 April 2022. The pieces are falling together. I have not been keeping up my journal as so much has happened and things to do. I came back from a weekend getaway to visit Jackie in February to be greeted with the news that my friend and neighbor's husband passed away from his illness. He had suffered for a while and the Lord decided to ease the pain. He and Gary were close and I debated as to whether to tell Gary or not, but every now and then he would ask about him, so I decided that honesty in this case was the best policy with him as he knew his friend was extremely ill. Gary took the news hard and commented on how he never expected to outlive him and wished he himself had never taken the chemotherapy treatments and just lived out his life with quality. Gary could tell I was upset and he asked me if I was o.k. I miss Gary so much and still love him so much it breaks my heart. Today is our 23rd anniversary and I had totally not registered it in my mind until my daughter mentioned it in our visit last week. Weird, but it is the 3rd wedding anniversary that he has not been at home with me.

I am always torn in my feelings when I prepare to visit – last year he had no clue but last weekend he seemed to be aware. I do not know if it was a "Lucky Day" or the Seroquel that they are finally giving him to help with the psychotic episodes. It is so stressful and tiring to visit. At least once I retire, I will have more flexibility when I can visit and hopefully the stress will be minimized.

1 April 2022

The Lord has provided grace to us with other family issues so we can be relieved and move forward. I am down to 15 working days left and I know the Lord will guide me to what and where I need to be for my next chapter – it is as exciting as it can get given the circumstances. I have not told Gary that I am retiring as I do not want him to get anxious, stressed or have expectations for me that I am not ready to deal with. Over time it will become apparent if he can put it together.

10 April 2022

My visit with Gary today was frustrating – he was in a very tired mode, not really with it at all and the rash on his legs are really ugly. The staff says they have much improved but I have to wonder what is going on in his body. He was in his needy mode today as well, which gets very frustrating – he wanted to go to a store, flea market, restaurants, etc. that I can not take him to and he gets testy with me. Anyway, the room was clean and he had his supplies so they are taking care of him properly. It is a shame that he will not be able to be active with me on the retirement journey – I had to work through his journey.

14 April 2022

Read something today that the harder your life is the bigger your God given purpose is – I hope that I fully understand the purpose soon.

25 April 2022

In addition to my visits with Gary I have had my retirement party. Nice and small as I requested. Life is weird – just like I knew the Lord called me to my current position I also know that the Lord is calling me to new challenges and a different way of life - ---

2 May 2022

Well, the last week has been a major deviation of what I thought would be happening. Last Thursday on my last morning at the office I was contacted by the hospital. Gary was admitted to the ER with what turned out to be a fatal intestinal evisceration. Gary was in a state of pain that forced him to scream and be pale. He knew death was coming. After a lot of discussions and issues we were able to get him on Hospice to end his pain. We told him it was o.k. to let go. I feel that he suffered enough to ask the Lord to take him and ensure his sins were forgiven – Christ knew he was a good man, and he was wanted at home. Another part of my plan is changing. I believe with every piece of my mind and body that God has an incredibly unique plan for me given the series of events and I just need to keep my mind open so I see the path when it is presented. Gary went to be with our Father in Heaven on 30 April, my official retirement date.

I am filled with a lot of mixed emotions – relief he is not suffering anymore, denial that we will not see him anymore, thankful to be unencumbered as I go into my next phase of life and thankful that I had his love for 26 years. It is a great feeling to have been so blessed with a great husband and father for my children.

6 May 2022

Today I cremated my husband, my love and my friend. It was an extremely difficult time but all three of us made it through. Lots of crying and saying our personal farewells. He was sent forth as the Gary we always knew groomed well, with green hair in his mohawk and dressed in the clothes he loved to wear, with a couple of his favorite items that were allowed. His days of watching the lumberjacks from his window were over and now he can look down from Heaven while he laughs and his angel wings protect them. If I am Blessed enough to have another man in my life he will truly have to be sent straight from God as no other will be worthy.

7 May 2022

The memorial service was beautiful. We took great care to ensure every detail reflected Gary and our love for him. All three of us presented eulogies and that process really helped us frame our love and journey that last three years. We were grateful when it was over, and we could all go to our personal spaces and really start processing any tears that remained and gain our focus to move back into life. R.I.P my husband, my love, my friend.

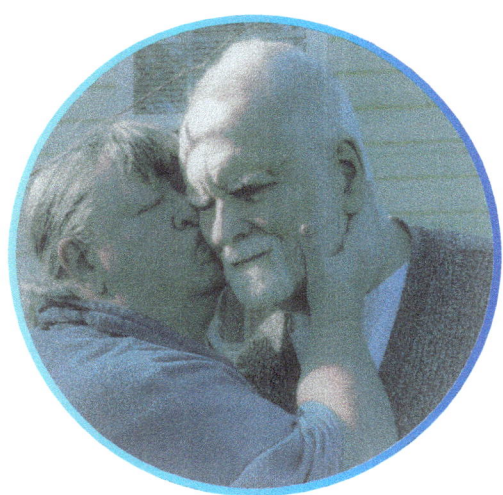

TIME TO HEAL, INTEGRATE INTO THE NEW PHASE OF LIFE AND DETERMINE THE PURPOSE THAT GOD FREED ME TO PURSUE.

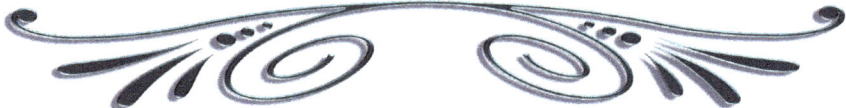

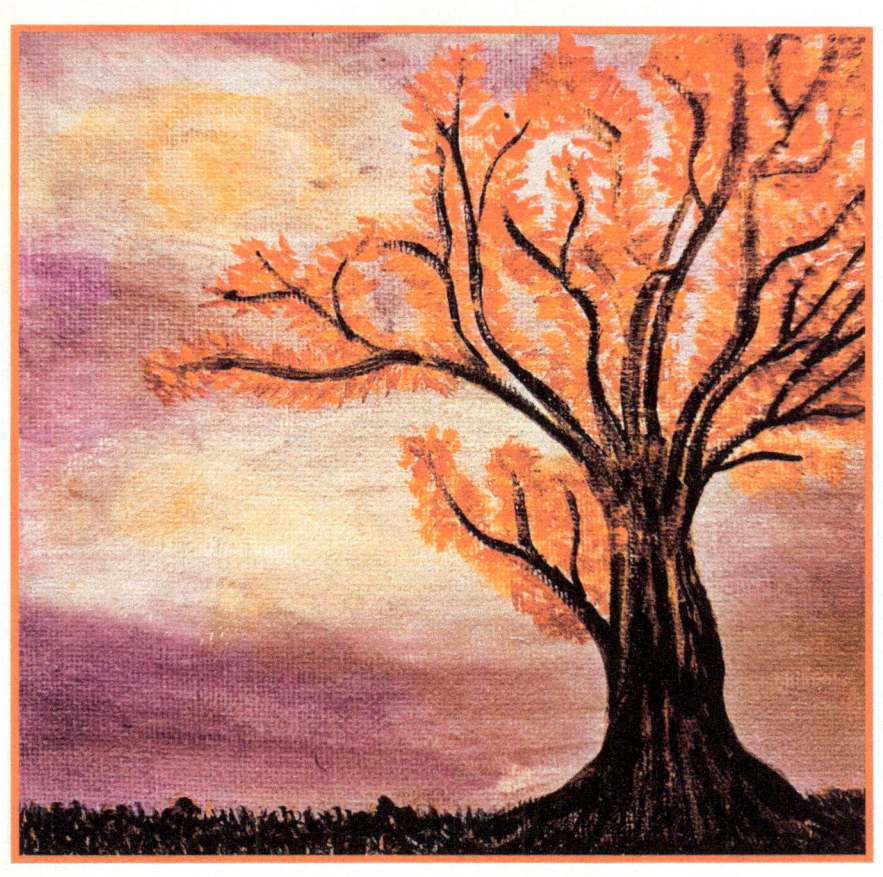

Tree Stands Alone

A NEW CHAPTER

Out of the darkness and into the light
No longer scared nor willing to take flight
You are always with me as my journey unfolds
Who knows what stories will get told
The "me" of the "them" will come into sight
God will make sure that everything is alright
It is time for the "me" to have a fresh start
Now is the time the "them" will forever be apart
I will see you in Heaven when God demands
Meanwhile I will have fun dancing in the sand!

EPILOGUE

As the sun sets over the lumberjack camp, he closes his eyes and starts to float away, watching the lumberjacks below go home to their families. Finally, free from confusion, fear, frustration and pain, he smiles, knowing he was well loved on this place called Earth and rises to the Gates of Heaven.

" He's a Lumberjack and he's o.k."

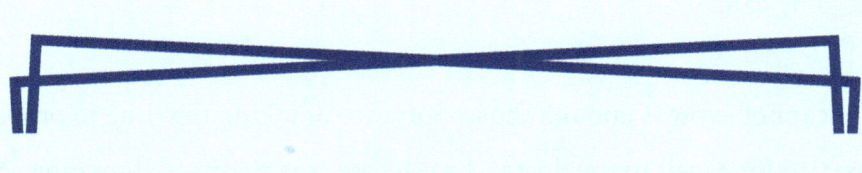

VISITATION/PREPARATION GUIDE

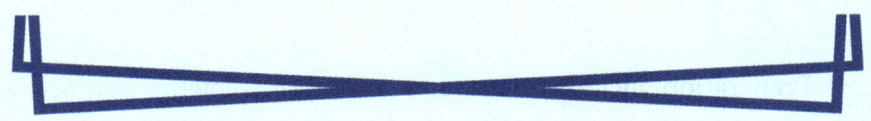

The best preparation is to have in place all legal documents for estate planning, health related decisions and power of attorney needs before you start treatments, have surgery or start to have memory issues. If not in place it can place an unforeseen tremendous burden on your loved ones if you are not capable of making decisions or pass away . If you are still healthy and can manage it financially, long-term care insurance is well worth the investment. The cost is reduced significantly the sooner you get it and will provide a blanket of financial security in the event you need ongoing care.

I cannot express enough the importance of taking the time to properly prepare for a visit to the doctor, health care treatments and memory care patients. There is so much that happens and is expected of you and the afflicted at these visits that you need to be shielded in strength to get through them. Your shield is developed through preparation.

Preparation includes, first and foremost, allowing yourself as a caregiver to do what you need in order to be emotionally, spiritually, mentally and physically able to perform the tasks required of you in a rational, efficient and safe manner. This will differ by person but will likely involve a routine or ritual of one or more of the following: rest, focus, worship, meditation, sleep, healthy eating and hydration, exercise, social interaction, hobbies, support groups, therapy, etc. Please make sure you allow for your self-care in this journey. Your ability to sustain any long-term caregiving for an illness requires you to be healthy.

VISITATION PREPARATION GUIDE / CHECKLIST

1. Create a space for yourself to be alone if you are living with others, so that you can be by yourself to process everything as needed. Where is your space?

2. Create a space to use for preparation of items for appointments, treatments and visits, so that you have a dedicated area and can have items handy for movement from one carry bag to another as needed. Define your space:

3. Duplicate some items like tissues, snacks, etc. so you don't have to always move things around if each event requires a lot of specialized items, but you also need basic supplies. What are your items?

4. It is important that if you have to wait or be in treatments for a long period of time to have a prepared healthy lunch, snacks, drinks, etc. What is your favorite allowed go-to foods?

5. Prepare for your and the patient's entertainment during the visits, crossword books, music lists with earbuds, reading books/magazines, crochet/knit, etc. What interests you and your loved one?

6. For memory care visits you need to plan even more for how you will interact and have a backup plan in case the visit is not going as you hope - memory books, crafts, balloon toss, storytelling, celebratory items or food, etc. Be willing to go with the flow and be imaginative as that can be the saving grace in your time with your loved one. What are your loved one's favorite things? What do they need to work on (physical or mental) exercises?

7. What supplies need to be replenished: medical supplies, grooming items, clothing, reading material, writing material, if permitted (note: pens, pencils can be weaponized and may not be permitted), slippers, towels, deodorizers, hangers, hampers, shower chairs, other furniture requirements, wall hangings, family photos, unbreakable handheld mirrors, tv's or music players if allowed, specialty items, etc. What are key items you know you need to bring regularly?

8. Make notes for what occurred during the visit and any items/questions/concerns that you need to pursue or bring next time.

Questions/Concerns for Preparation for Doctor and Treatment visits:

1. Talk about the duration in days, weeks, months of the treatment plan.

2. How long and often are treatments required? Each day, week, month, etc.

3. Side Effects that can be expected – understand the uncommon ones as well, you could be the minority percentage.

4. Transportation concerns…

5. Who is available for support during your visits (if you attend by yourself, who is your emergency point of contact)?

6. Quality of life issues (really research what is being suggested for you to see if the plan fits in with how you want to live your life).

7. Ensure your legal paperwork is in order (wills, living wills, advanced medical directives, Power of Attorney, do not resuscitate, trusts, etc.) This cannot be under emphasized – be prepared.

8. Rehabilitation requirements – understand the known requirements and length, so barring any unforeseen issues, you can have a facility already picked out and scheduled for any post treatment/surgery needs.

9. Do research on the hospital / treatment facility to ensure it fits your needs and specializes in the care you require.

10. Do some financial planning for any missed income during your recovery.

11. Who will be staying with you during recovery, if needed

12. What are your dietary restrictions?11. Sometimes it is temporary, sometimes it is permanent. Understand your post illness needs to remain healthy.

13. What medical equipment, special needs will you require. This is important as you may have to rearrange your living environment or schedule to accommodate on going life sustaining issues, temporarily or on a permanent basis.

14. How much does your insurance cover for pre, during, post and ongoing needs for treatments, surgery, rehabilitation, recovery and ongoing health maintenance?

15. What are your spiritual, emotional and mental support needs during these periods of time? Ensure you have a plan in place to have those needs met and that your loved ones understand your desires.

16. Provide a framework if not a prearranged plan for any funeral and bequeath wishes, just in case.

There are likely other items that your particular situation may require, but these are the basics.

Proper planning allows for the patient and loved ones to understand and process more of the situation they are going to be experiencing, potentially reducing the level of stress.

The following pages are intentionally left blank for space to document any thoughts, details or plans. A companion journal is also available.

www.ingramcontent.com/pod-product-compliance
Lightning Source LLC
Chambersburg PA
CBHW070617030426
42337CB00020B/3835